# Medicines Management for Nurses at a Glance

This title is also available as an e-book.
For more details, please see
**www.wiley.com/buy/9781118840726**
or scan this QR code:

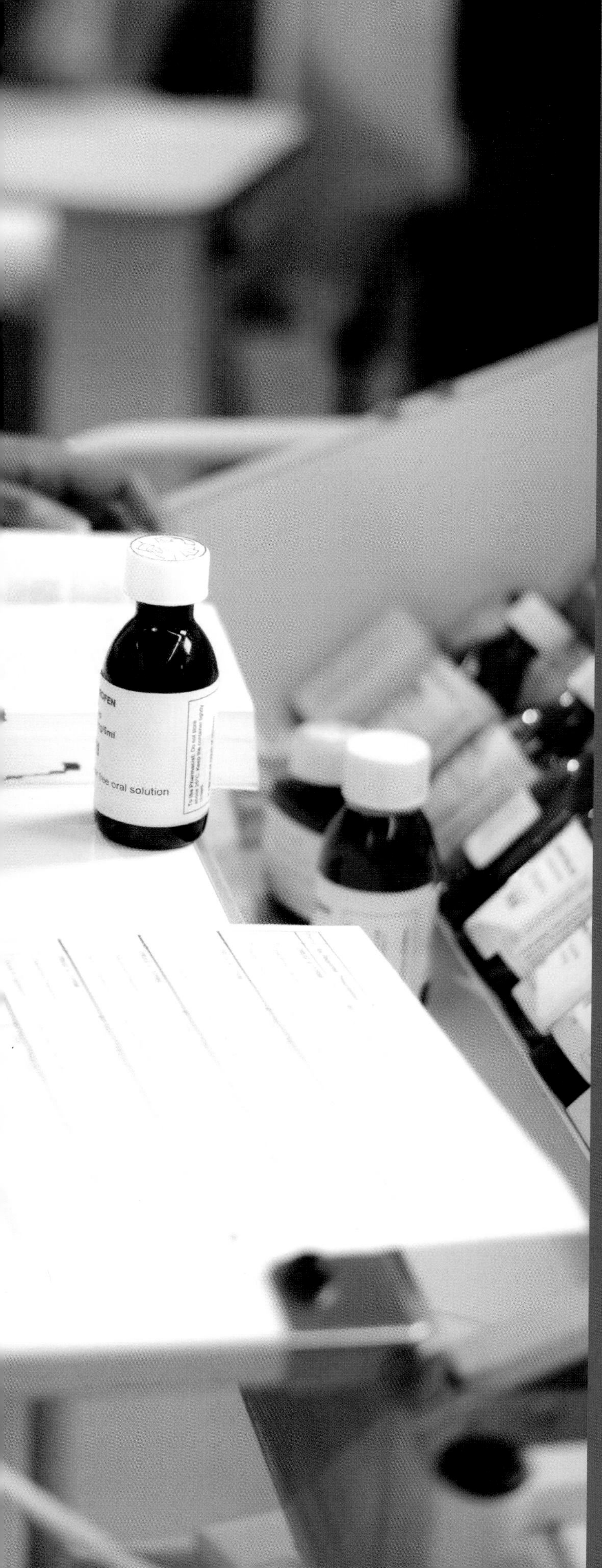

# Medicines Management for Nurses at a Glance

**Simon Young**
Academic Subject Manager – Medicines Management and Prescribing
Faculty of Life Sciences and Education
University of South Wales

**Ben Pitcher**
Senior Lecturer
Faculty of Life Sciences and Education
University of South Wales

**Series editor: Ian Peate**

WILEY Blackwell

*Registered office:* John Wiley & Sons, Ltd, The Atrium, Southern Gate, Chichester, West Sussex, PO19 8SQ, UK

*Editorial offices:* 9600 Garsington Road, Oxford, OX4 2DQ, UK
The Atrium, Southern Gate, Chichester, West Sussex, PO19 8SQ, UK
350 Main Street, Malden, MA 02148-5020, USA

For details of our global editorial offices, for customer services and for information about how to apply for permission to reuse the copyright material in this book please see our website at www.wiley.com/wiley-blackwell



***Library of Congress Cataloging-in-Publication Data***

Young, Simon, 1971- , author.
Medicines management for nurses at a glance / Simon Young, Ben Pitcher.
p. ; cm. – (At a glance series)
Includes index.
ISBN 978-1-118-84072-6 (paperback)
I. Pitcher, Ben, 1979-, author. II. Title. III. Series: At a glance series (Oxford, England)
[DNLM: 1. Drug Therapy–nursing–Great Britain. 2. Drug Prescriptions–nursing–Great Britain. 3. Drug Therapy–methods–Great Britain. 4. Nurse Clinicians–Great Britain. WY 100 FA1]
RT68
615.1'4–dc23

2015033805

A catalogue record for this book is available from the British Library.

Wiley also publishes its books in a variety of electronic formats. Some content that appears in print may not be available in electronic books.

Cover image: GettyImages-478860007/sturti

Set in 9.5/11.5pt Minion Pro by Aptara, India
Printed and bound in Singapore by Markono Print Media Pte Ltd

1 2016

# Contents

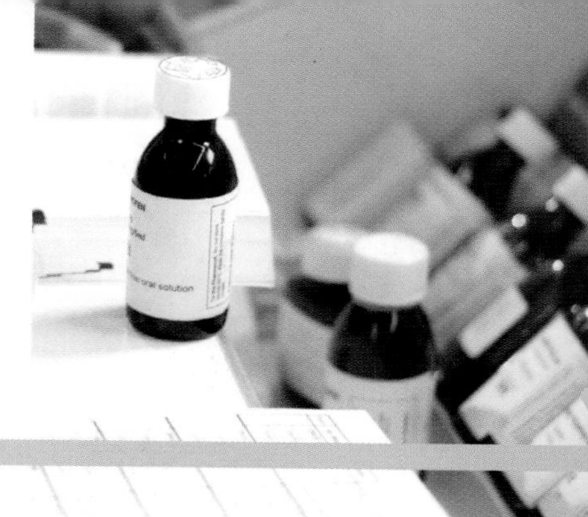

## Part 3 Safe and effective medicines management 89

# Preface

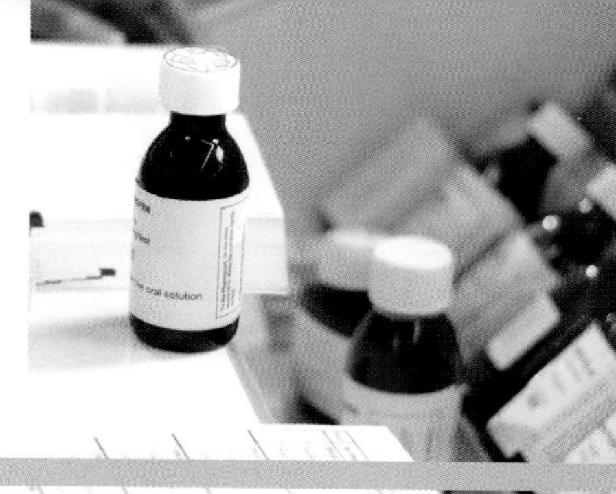

The main aims of this publication are twofold: to introduce pre-registration nursing students to the principles of managing medicines and to aid more experienced nurses (and other healthcare professionals) to develop a better sense of the breadth and depth of medicines management.

In order that standards of teaching and learning and curriculum delivery are equitably set across all universities, the Nursing and Midwifery Council (NMC) oversees the accreditation of nursing curricula. Despite this, there will be varying emphasis on the importance of each of the many subject areas that make up the knowledge base of nursing. The nurse's knowledge of pharmacology will vary significantly for a variety of reasons. Many nurses will not have formally studied pharmacological science in their training and we hope this book will offer a gateway to pharmacological knowledge, which is key to managing medicines.

Many pharmacology texts consider the subject in great depth and offer insight into the development of basic pharmacological science through to complex evidence-based clinical pharmacology. This book attempts to look directly at pharmacology, and its impact on clinical practice and on managing medicines safely and efficaciously. It often refers to the important cardinal resources of medicines management such as the British National Formulary (BNF), the NMC standards and the summary of product characteristics (SPC) of the medicine. These resources should be read alongside this text to gain further perspective on the use of medicines in modern health care. The text does not aim to replace these resources but we hope it will assist in understanding their importance and offer critical consideration of their use. In addition the book, while accurate and up to date, does not replace guidelines, protocols and other evidence-based texts. Professional judgement and up to date knowledge should always be applied in making clinical decisions directly affecting the health and well-being of patients.

The book covers a range of topics and is **not** designed for one branch or field of nursing practice. A range of fundamental medicines management principles and therapeutic topics are considered and explored. For example, chapters tackling substance misuse should be relevant to most areas of practice but will be more applicable and practically useful to some specific branches of nursing. The size of the '… at a glance' books means that some topics we wanted to cover didn't make the cut. The presence or absence of a topic does not reflect upon the importance of that topic. The topics selected afforded us, as authors, an opportunity to encourage readers to consider applying principles learned to other areas of medicines management.

The charts seen in the therapeutic topics sections are variations of the 'prescription charts' seen in hospitals or Medicines Administration Record Sheets seen in care home settings. The lessons learned from these topics apply to managing those medicines across **all** areas of practice (e.g. in community-based settings). The charts enabled us to share some practical knowledge with regards medicines to administration and management that add value and authenticity to the text.

Throughout the book we have used the terms 'nurse' and 'healthcare professional'. We acknowledge that the term 'nurse' could be replaced by the term 'midwife' but for brevity we have used the term 'nurse'. In, addition we have used the term 'patient' most often to refer to the person who is taking the medication. We appreciate that terminology varies from practice area to practice area and acknowledge that 'patients' are people - just like us. We use the term 'patient' not to define the person but to define the responsibility the healthcare professional has for their care. This book, it is hoped, will contribute to a better understanding of medicines and the people who take them. We hope that in some way it will also contribute something positive to managing medicines and to the people who take them.

Finally, Ben and I would like to offer our thanks to those who have supported us in putting this book together. First, we would like to thank the team at Wiley, especially Karen and James, for their dedication, patience and support.  Second, we would like to thank all the patients, students and healthcare professionals who have inspired us as practising healthcare professionals and educators. The last and most important thanks go to our families. Special thanks go to our wives, Jess and Tash, who offered us so much support through the entire process. An additional thanks to our inspirational offspring: Jack, Jacob, Lily, Luke and Lydia – this book would not have been possible without you.

Ben Pitcher and
Simon Young

# About the companion website

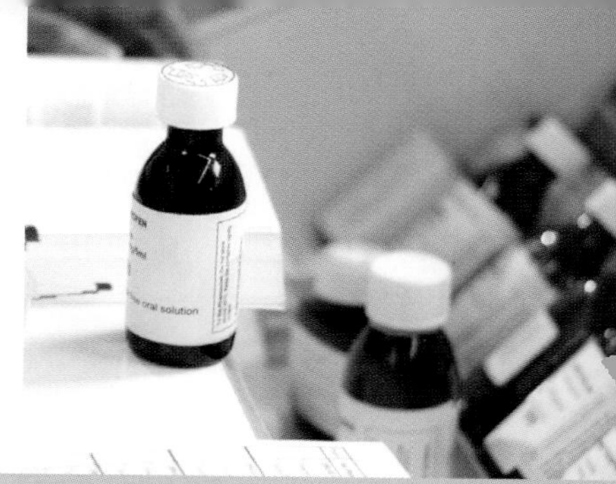

Don't forget to visit the companion website for this book:

**ataglanceseries.com/nursing/medicinesmanagement**

There you will find valuable material designed to enhance your learning, including:

- Interactive multiple choice questions

Scan this QR code to visit the companion website

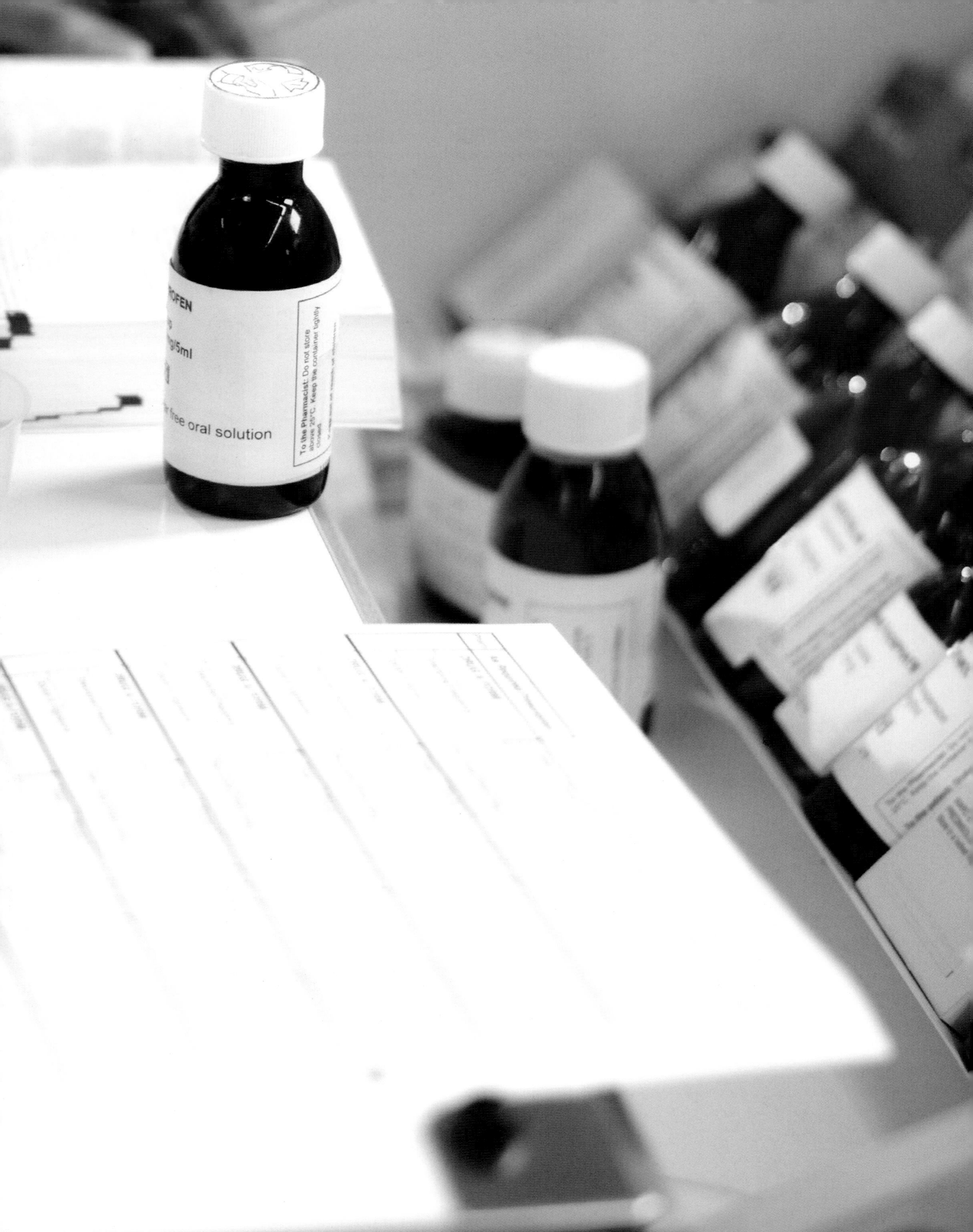
free oral solution
To the Pharmacist: Do not store above 25°C. Keep the container tightly closed.

# Introduction to pharmacology and medicines management

## Chapters

# 1 Why is managing medicines important in nursing?

**Figure 1.1** An overlapping Venn diagram illustrating the Nursing and Midwifery Council's elements of the medicines management skills cluster

## Medicines management and nursing

Nursing is a multifaceted profession. A wide variety of knowledge and skills is required to become a safe and effective nurse in modern healthcare practice. The essential skills clusters (ESCs) of the Nursing and Midwifery Council (NMC) define and illustrate the essential skills that are to be developed by the pre-registration nurse to make that nurse fit for registration. The NMC has developed five clusters of knowledge and skills related to nursing competence:

- Care, compassion and communication.
- Organisational aspects of care.
- Infection prevention and control.
- Nutrition and fluid management.
- Medicines management.

This book will focus on the medicines management cluster and explore the important medicines-related knowledge required by a nurse. Whenever possible, the ESC will be referenced so that you may consider your knowledge and skill development in that area of medicines management as you work through the book.

## Defining medicines management

The Audit Commission report, 'A Spoonful of Sugar: Medicines Management in NHS Hospitals' (2001), was designed to highlight the importance of the effective use of medication as a part of the nurse's role. While nurses' involvement with medicines management varies according to the context of care (e.g. community based, hospital based), the report highlights that up to '7,000 individual doses are administered daily in a "typical" hospital; and up to 40 per cent of nurses' time is spent administering medicines' (http://www.eprescribingtoolkit.com/wp-content/uploads/2013/11/nrspoonfulsugar1.pdf, point 11, p.9, last accessed 6 August, 2015).

The report defined medicines management as:

> *Medicines management in hospitals encompasses the entire way that medicines are selected, procured, delivered, prescribed, administered and reviewed to optimise the contribution that medicines make to producing informed and desired outcomes of patient care.*
>
> (www.eprescribingtoolkit.com/wp-content/uploads/2013/11/nrspoonfulsugar1.pdf, Box A, p.5, last accessed 6 August, 2015)

This definition illustrates that managing medicines is not just the responsibility of pharmacists and doctors. It is the collective responsibility of those who work for a healthcare organisation. When working in the NHS, it is easy to find examples of nurses who undertake every facet of medicines management (Figure 1.1). Nurses commonly prescribe, dispense, administer and review patient medication on a day-to-day basis.

The report continues by identifying the main reasons why medicines management needs to continually improve. Medication errors are unacceptably common, the efficacy of medicines is increasing, the costs of medicines are rising and the administration of medicines is becoming more complex. In addition, there is a need to review medicines management across whole health economies as the distinction between primary and secondary care becomes increasingly blurred.

Managing medicines is more than just clinical pharmacology. Clinical pharmacological knowledge is an essential element of safe and efficacious patient care along with the other core skills.

Figure 1.1 is not hierarchical but attempts to illustrate the interconnected nature of the ESCs that make up the medicines management process. Understanding how medicines work (their fundamental pharmacology) is significant knowledge in, for example, medicines administration. Understanding fundamental pharmacokinetics (Chapters 6 and 7) and fundamental pharmacodynamics (Chapters 10 and 11) allow the nurse undertaking medication administration to explain the dose of medication prescribed, its clinical indication, its likely beneficial effects and any potentially important adverse effects such as side effects (Chapter 48) and drug interactions (Chapter 47).

Traditionally, doctors prescribe, pharmacists dispense and nurses administer medication. Modern healthcare practice incorporates increasingly diverse means of supplying medicine: there are growing numbers of prescribers from a range of professional backgrounds (nurses, pharmacists and physiotherapists) and additional ways for patients to access medication – for example, patient group directions (PGDs), which are written instructions for the supply or administration of medicines to groups of patients according to a set of predetermined criteria. The competent nurse needs to understand their role in supporting these mechanisms of medicine supply and in facilitating patient access to increasingly complex treatments as part of evidence-based interventions.

Economic predictions of the cost of medicines in the UK reached a figure in excess of £15 billion by 2015. A proportion of these medicines are established interventions for frequently occurring conditions that reflect the general ill health of the nation. However, some of the costs relate to newer pharmacotherapeutic innovations. Many medications currently used are aimed at preventing the serious consequences of untreated pathophysiological states (e.g. treating hypertension to prevent the cardiovascular consequences of the condition). This presents the NHS with a challenging future with regard to medicines selection and use. Increasingly, medicines use in practice is guided by nationally generated evidence such as National Institute for Health and Care Excellence (NICE) guidelines and technology appraisals. Royal Colleges and collectives such as the Faculty of Sexual and Reproductive Health also produce useful guidance with regard to medicines management. More and more, these guidelines are forming the fundamental basis for medicines choice in practice. Their aim is to ensure the equitable treatment of patients, and that the benefits to patients are optimised and the risks minimised.

The philosophy of managing medicines is increasingly attempting to engage patients in medication choice. Much of the guidance that relates, for example, to medicines choice in mental health aims to put the patient at the centre when selecting pharmacotherapies. In so doing, the aspiration is that adherence (the extent to which patients take medication as prescribed by healthcare professionals) will be increased.

Providing truly holistic care in nursing practice means appreciating both the art and the science of managing medicines.

# 2 Keeping up to date with medicines management

**Figure 2.1** An example of how even widely used medications can have significant changes in usage over time

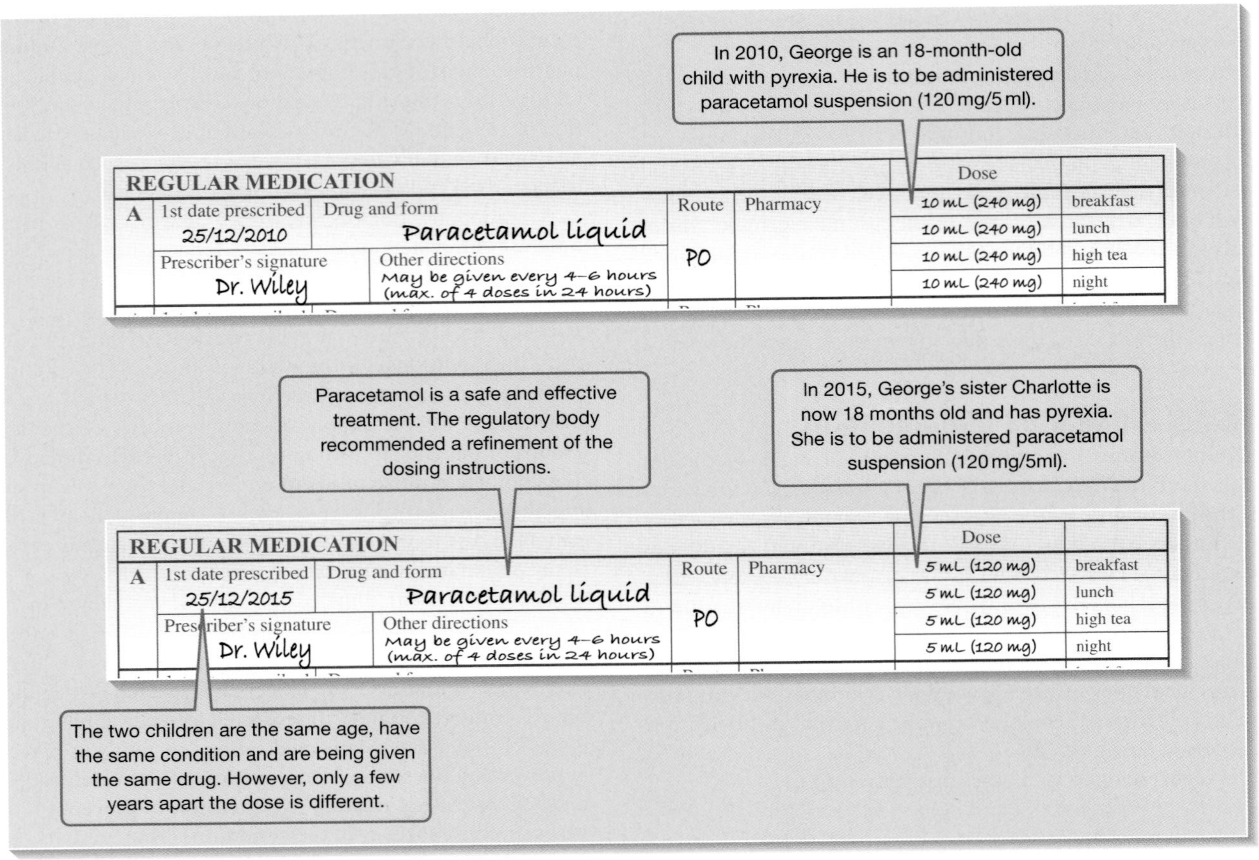

In 2010, George is an 18-month-old child with pyrexia. He is to be administered paracetamol suspension (120 mg/5 ml).

| REGULAR MEDICATION | | | | | Dose | |
|---|---|---|---|---|---|---|
| A | 1st date prescribed: 25/12/2010 | Drug and form: Paracetamol liquid | Route: PO | Pharmacy | 10 mL (240 mg) | breakfast |
| | Prescriber's signature: Dr. Wiley | Other directions: May be given every 4–6 hours (max. of 4 doses in 24 hours) | | | 10 mL (240 mg) | lunch |
| | | | | | 10 mL (240 mg) | high tea |
| | | | | | 10 mL (240 mg) | night |

Paracetamol is a safe and effective treatment. The regulatory body recommended a refinement of the dosing instructions.

In 2015, George's sister Charlotte is now 18 months old and has pyrexia. She is to be administered paracetamol suspension (120 mg/5ml).

| REGULAR MEDICATION | | | | | Dose | |
|---|---|---|---|---|---|---|
| A | 1st date prescribed: 25/12/2015 | Drug and form: Paracetamol liquid | Route: PO | Pharmacy | 5 mL (120 mg) | breakfast |
| | Prescriber's signature: Dr. Wiley | Other directions: May be given every 4–6 hours (max. of 4 doses in 24 hours) | | | 5 mL (120 mg) | lunch |
| | | | | | 5 mL (120 mg) | high tea |
| | | | | | 5 mL (120 mg) | night |

The two children are the same age, have the same condition and are being given the same drug. However, only a few years apart the dose is different.

## Continuing professional development

### Limitations of this book

As titled, this book is a glance at some fundamentals of medicines management. As such, it cannot be considered all that you need to know. Even learning everything in this book would only provide you with the most basic elements of medicines management. It is essential that practitioners continue to develop their knowledge and understanding of medications and pharmacology (Figure 2.1).

### Medicines administration

When administering drugs to patients, we must take steps to check that we are administering the drugs correctly. These are often described as the 5 'Rs' of drug administration:

- Right patient.
- Right drug.
- Right dose.
- Right route.
- Right time.

However, it is possible to complete this check list without fully understanding what the drug is and what it does.

### What does the Nursing and Midwifery Council say?

The Nursing and Midwifery Council (NMC) gives practitioners important guidance regarding the administration of medications. Included in this are statements as to what a practitioner should know about the pharmacology of drugs when administering them to patients: *'You must know the therapeutic uses of the medicine to be administered, its normal dosage, side effects, precautions and contra-indications'* (http://www.cmft.nhs.uk/media/299673/nmc%20standards%20for%20medicines%20management%20booklet.pdf, section 4, p. 7, last accessed 6 August, 2015).

This is the key statement. It highlights the depth of knowledge required by practitioners.

#### Therapeutic uses

It is not enough to simply administer a prescribed drug without knowing what it is for, trusting that the prescriber has made the appropriate choice. It is essential that you understand what the drug is for, to identify whether a prescribing error has been made (and they do occasionally happen).

#### Normal dosage

Knowing what the normal dosage is for a drug is an important way of preventing the over- or under-dosing of patients.

#### Side effects

Because many drugs have side effects, it is important to understand what these are so that you can identify them and act accordingly.

#### Precautions and contra-indications

It is important that you understand what precautions and contra-indications exist for a drug – that is, what conditions or comorbidities a patient might have that would make giving a certain drug inadvisable or even dangerous: *'You must administer or withhold in the context of the patient's condition'* (http://www.cmft.nhs.uk/media/299673/nmc%20standards%20for%20medicines%20management%20booklet.pdf, section 4, p. 7, last accessed 6 August, 2015).

This is another important concept for a practitioner to understand, building on the idea in the previous statement. A drug may have been prescribed to a patient by a doctor, and at the time it was prescribed everything was correct. However, it is possible that a change in the condition of the patient will mean that the drug may no longer be appropriate to administer. For example, the NMC advises that digoxin (an antiarrhythmic) should not usually be given to patients with a pulse rate lower than 60. An understanding of digoxin's action in lowering heart rate can help you identify this and avoid harming a patient. Another example would include withholding antiglycaemic drugs from diabetic patients who are already hypoglycaemic.

### Where to learn?

There is a lot to learn about medicines management. It is important to realise that memorising details about drugs has limited benefit because the details may change. The only answer is to stay up to date with the drugs that you commonly use, and to rely upon the tools that are available.

The **British National Formulary** (BNF; https://www.evidence.nhs.uk/formulary/bnf/current, last accessed 18 September, 2015) is an essential tool for all practitioners. It is the repository of information for nearly all drugs used in British health care. It is a tool you should become intimately familiar with, and make your first port of call regarding queries about drugs.

The **electronic Medicines Compendium** (eMC; http://www.medicines.org.uk/emc, last accessed 6 August, 2015) is a collection of summaries of product characteristics (SPCs) and patient information leaflets (PILs). These are a useful resource and often contain details not found in the BNF.

The National Institute for Health and Care Excellence (NICE) **medicines optimisation guidelines** (http://www.nice.org.uk/guidance/ng5, last accessed 6 August, 2015) provide information on how to use medications in the safest and most effective way, reduce harm and ensure patient benefit.

### The evolving evidence base

A new edition of the printed BNF is published every 6 months. The BNF online is updated more frequently. This is due in part to the new drugs being developed and the continual evolution of the safe use of medicines.

We refer to health care as being evidence based. The actions we take and the drugs we administer are determined by evidence derived from research. However, research is not done once and then never re-examined: it is an ongoing process. Our understanding of therapy and conditions will change over time. For example, recommended doses can change, and new side effects and contra-indications can be discovered. Practitioners must keep learning to keep up to date.

## Post-registration educational practice

The NMC requires practitioners to undertake post-registration education and practice (Prep). Once qualified, a nurse does not leave learning and study behind. They must continue to expand their knowledge and skills, and keep the ones they have up to date.

While medicines management is not the only area that needs to be continually updated, it is an important one. Take time to learn about the drugs used in your area. When new drugs are introduced, read about them in the BNF, download the SPCs and talk to prescribers about how the drugs are used. All this learning can be kept and explored by using reflective practice. Through this, you can build a portfolio of learning that can be used as evidence for your employer and your regulatory body.

# What is a medicine?

**Figure 3.1** The stages of development of a new medicine from new chemical entity to the patient. The numbers are approximate and demonstrate the effort, investment and time required to develop a new drug. Healthcare professionals are primarily involved in the final section (green) and will have significant influence over the success of the product

| Phase | Pre-discovery phase | Drug discovery | Pre-clinical work | Clinical trials | | | Regulatory approval | Marketing and post-marketing surveillance |
|---|---|---|---|---|---|---|---|---|
| Number of compounds (candidates) | | 10,000 or more | 250 compounds | 5–10 | <5 | <5 | 1 | 1 |
| Time taken | | 3–6 years | | 6–7 years | | | 0.5–2 years | |
| | | | | Phase I | Phase II | Phase III | Review and approval | |
| Number of volunteers | | | | 20–100 | 100–500 | 1000–5000 | Eligible patient population | |
| Description of activity in each phase | These phases include:<br>• Understanding the disease and its biochemistry<br>• Identifying targets, e.g. genes and receptors and screening compounds for that target.<br>This will lead to identifying the best compound (often termed a candidate drug).<br>Pre-clinical testing includes safety evaluation, trial design and manufacturing sufficient candidate compound. | | | Early clinical trials and non-clinical studies aim to confirm what earlier studies have shown. The focus here is on how the candidate behaves in humans not in the laboratory:<br>**Phase I** consists of collecting data on the basic pharmacology of the drug and its safety in healthy volunteers.<br>**Phase II** studies are undertaken on those who have the target condition the drug will eventually treat when marketed. This phase establishes dose ranges and the drug's efficacy and safety in a patient sub-population.<br>**Phase III** is similar to Phase II but larger in scale and data are gathered to provide evidence to the regulatory authority that will grant the manufacturer the right to market the drug. | | | Research data are submitted to the regulatory agencies (worldwide) and the medication may then be marketed.<br>Post-marketing surveillance takes place. | |

Defining the word 'medicine' is not as simple as it first seems. There is a bewildering array of products found in hospital and community nursing practice that are used to treat and prevent illness. Practitioners and patients alike will use terms such as 'medication', 'medicines', 'pills' and 'drugs' without considering what connotations these words have to those around them.

'Medicines' is a term that is generally used for drugs that have been prepared for administration to humans or animals (Figure 3.1). By this definition, the aspirin powder that is found in a factory awaiting formulation into a tablet is a **drug** and the aspirin tablets that are manufactured and then administered to patients are **medicines** or **medicinal products**.

The term 'drug' is used in practice when referring to a 'drug round' or 'drug trolley'. This is common healthcare nomenclature but the term 'drug' has negative connotations such as 'drug abuse', 'drug dealer' and 'drug smuggling'. Taking care to use the appropriate terminology is important in inspiring confidence in patients that their medication is efficacious and will have the desired therapeutic benefit.

The Human Medicines Regulations 2012 define a 'medicinal product' as:

*(a) any substance or combination of substances presented as having properties of preventing or treating disease in human beings; or*

*(b) any substance or combination of substances that may be used by or administered to human beings with a view to—*

*(i) restoring, correcting or modifying a physiological function by exerting a pharmacological, immunological or metabolic action, or*

*(ii) making a medical diagnosis.*

(http://www.legislation.gov.uk/uksi/2012/1916/pdfs/uksi_20121916_en.pdf, accessed 6 August, 2015)

This definition appears very technical and is designed to clarify what could be characterised as a medicine by the law in Great Britain. It acts as a starting point for an Act of Parliament that defines how medicines are (among other things) manufactured, bought and sold, dispensed and administered.

The definition probably bears some resemblance to the definition of a medicine that you may have in mind. When reading the features of medicinal products, you will start to recognise the features of medicines encountered in clinical practice. Some medicines modify physiological functions (e.g. diuretics) while others replace deficiencies of substances that would normally be found in the body (e.g. iron supplements). Some drugs prevent illness (e.g. the measles, mumps and rubella [MMR] vaccine) while others have no direct effect on the body but aid diagnosis (e.g. Gastrografin®). It is important to note that the Human Medicines Regulations and their definitions do not include whole blood or blood products (unless industrially manufactured). The use of these products is covered by other legislation and while they appear to be used in the same way as medicines, they are not legally defined in the same way.

When considering the meaning of the term 'medicine', it is important to consider the patient's perspective of medicines. When taking a medication history from a patient, note that some will not consider their inhalers to be medicines. Many will visit alternative or complementary practitioners (e.g. a homeopath or herbalist) and not necessarily consider the remedies prescribed by those practitioners as medicines. There are many products that may fit the definition of a medicine as outlined earlier but are not treated as medicines from a legal perspective. Antiperspirants arguably 'modify physiological function' but their manufacture is not covered by medicines legislation. However, Driclor® is technically an antiperspirant that is a medicinal product because it is used to treat the condition known as hyperhidrosis. Many vitamins and supplement products also fit the bill but their manufacture is governed by food legislation (unless the product has an identified medicinal purpose).

Patients may also take recreational drugs (both legal and illegal) and these form an important part in understanding the patient's perspective on drugs and the role they play in influencing health and well-being. Often, despite advice to the contrary from healthcare professionals, well-meaning patients share prescription only and pharmacy category (Chapter 50) medicines. A logical and caring perspective on these aspects of what defines a medicine assists in good medicines management practice.

## How are medicines developed and monitored?

The process of the development of new medicines is outlined in Figure 3.1. Built into this and the subsequent process of the ongoing manufacture of medicines are the three pillars of the pharmaceutical good manufacturing process: safety, quality and efficacy.

The development process, and its inbuilt quality control and assurance, ensures that healthcare professionals can make the most accurate and safe decisions with regard to medicines selection for patients. These processes accurately define the key features of medicines use such as route of administration (tablets, capsules, suppositories, etc.), the total daily dose, the dosing interval and the patient monitoring required. The initial side effect profiles and medication interactions associated with the medication are also uncovered. These features govern the practice of healthcare professionals associated with prescribing, dispensing and administering medication, and are important features of the essential skills clusters (ESCs) defined by the Nursing and Midwifery Council (NMC).

When medicines reach the stage when they are marketed (green column in Figure 3.1), it is a requirement that they are monitored to ensure that they continue to be suitable for use. The process of pharmacovigilance takes place and the use of medicines in a large population of patients is monitored. This ensures a medication's ongoing efficacy and safety.

The process of developing medicines, from the laboratory tests that define their pharmacology to reaching a population of patients, is costly in terms of both time and finance. Medicines management by nurses sits at the end of this process. Nurses, in their role of patient advocate, hold the key to ensuring that the patients' view of medicines is fair, balanced and evidence based.

# 4 Medicines nomenclature: what's in a name?

**Figure 4.1** An example of a drug monograph from the BNF. The monograph illustrates a range of information including the generic/approved name of the drug (Fluoxetine) and the brand/trade name (Prozac®). Source: *British National Formulary (BNF)*

**FLUOXETINE**

***Additional information*** interactions (Fluoxetine).

**Indications** see under Dose

**Cautions** see *notes above*

**Contra-indications** see *notes above*

**Hepatic impairment** reduce dose or increase dose interval

**Pregnancy** see *notes above*

**Breast-feeding** present in milk – avoid

**Side-effects** see *notes above*; also diarrhoea, dysphagia, vasodilatation, hypotension, flushing, palpation, pharyngitis, dyspnoea, chills, taste disturbance, sleep disturbances, malaise, euphoria, confusion, yawning, impaired concentration, changes in blood sugar, alopecia, urinary frequency; haemorrhage, pulmonary inflammation and fibrosis, hepatitis, toxic epidermal necrolysis, priapism, and neuroleptic malignant syndrome-like event also reported

**Dose**

- Major depression, 20 mg daily increased after 3–4 weeks if necessary, and at appropriate intervals thereafter; max. 60 mg daily (**elderly** usual max. 40 mg daily but 60 mg can be used); **child** 8–18 years, 10 mg daily increased after 1–2 weeks if necessary, max. 20 mg daily (but see also **Depressive Illness in Children and Adolescents**)
- Bulimia nervosa, **adult** over 18 years, 60 mg daily as a single or divided dose (**elderly** usual max. 40 mg daily but 60 mg can be used)
- Obsessive-compulsive disorder, **adult** over 18 years, 20 mg daily; increased gradually if necessary to max. 60 mg daily (**elderly** usual max. 40 mg daily but 60mg can be used); review treatment if inadequate response after 10 weeks

**Note** – Daily dose may be administered as a single or divided dose

**Long duration of action** – Consider the long half-life of fluoxetine when adjusting dosage (or in overdosage)

**Preparations**

Fluoxetine

**Prozac® (Lilly)**

**Capsules**, fluoxetine (as hydrochloride) 20 mg (green/yellow), net price 30-cap pack = £1.50. Counselling, driving

**Liquid**, fluoxetine (as hydrochloride) 20 mg/5mL, net price 70 mL = £11.12. Counselling, driving

**Figure 4.2** The non-proprietary and brand names applied to fluoxetine in the BNF

| Non-proprietary (or generic) name | Brand (or trade) name |
|---|---|
| Fluoxetine | Prozac® |

**Figure 4.3** The non-proprietary, brand and chemical names of two commonly used medicines

| Non-proprietary (or generic) name | Brand (or trade) name | Chemical name |
|---|---|---|
| Fluoxetine | Prozac® | N-methyl-3-phenyl-3-[4-(trifluoromethyl)phenoxy]propan-1-amine |
| Paracetamol | Panadol® | N-acetyl-para-aminophenol |

**Figure 4.4** Examples of medicines belonging to the phenothiazine family

| Medication name | | |
|---|---|---|
| **Non-proprietary name** | **Trade name** | **Example of use in clinical practice (BNF classification)** |
| Chlorpromazine | Largactil® | Antipsychotic |
| Prochlorperazine | Stemetil® | Nausea and vertigo |
| Levomepromazine | Nozinan® | Nausea and vertigo |
| Fluphenazine | Modecate® | Antipsychotic |

**Figure 4.5** Commonly used medicine name suffixes

| Suffix | Medication family or class | Examples |
|---|---|---|
| **-mab** | Monoclonal antibodies | Trastuzumab (used in chemotherapy) |
| **-olol** | β blockers | Propranolol and bisoprolol |
| **-sartan** | Angiotensin receptor antagonists | Valsartan |
| **-pril** | Angiotensin-converting enzyme inhibitors | Lisinopril and ramipril |
| **-cillin** | Penicillin antibiotics | Penicillin and amoxicillin |

*Medicines Management for Nurses at a Glance*. First Edition. Simon Young and Ben Pitcher. 
www.ataglanceseries.com/nursing/medicinesmanagement

One of the challenges faced by a healthcare professional is to develop a knowledge and understanding of medicines, their names and how they are used in everyday practice.

Figure 4.1 is an extract from the electronic version of the British National Formulary (BNF) providing important information for the use of fluoxetine. Clinically relevant details are included about the medicine (e.g. its recognised names, side effects, contraindications and dosing information). In the BNF there is an entry like this for every drug licensed for use in the UK. Each entry is called a 'monograph'.

The medication has two names in the BNF: fluoxetine (which can be found at the top of the monograph) and Prozac® (which is under the section called 'Preparations'). Fluoxetine is the 'non-proprietary' or 'generic' name. This is the name most commonly used in practice and most commonly seen on prescriptions and medication charts and in policies and guidelines.

Many medicines have 'brand' or 'trade' names. These are usually names that are given to the medication by their original manufacturer. These names uniquely identify a manufacturer's product including any particulars of the preparation (e.g. see Figure 4.2: Prozac® is the name of the fluoxetine preparation made by Lilly, who originally brought the medication to the market).

In general, the generic name should always be used when administering or prescribing a drug. However, when there is an established difference in clinical response between different brands of a medicine (usually noted in the BNF or in information provided by the manufacturer) a specific brand name should be used. An important example is the use of medicines that have a 'slow release', 'modified release' or 'controlled release' mechanism for delivering the active ingredient. Medicines like these often have specific features that mean the drug is released in a controlled fashion into the bloodstream. Swapping from one brand of medicines to another in this case is not always advisable. Differences in the specific characteristics of two different brands may result in a change in the speed with which the drug reaches the patient's blood. It may also influence the amount of drug absorbed, which may result in an unwanted variation in the patient's clinical response. The other most common reason for brand prescribing would be in the case of a drug with a narrow therapeutic index, such as products containing lithium or theophylline. Switching brands in this instance may lead to either a sub-therapeutic level of drug in the blood or an increased risk of toxicity and side effects. In this case it is very important that healthcare professionals ensure that the patient always receive the same branded product.

The use of the non-proprietary name in prescribing is usually the more cost-effective: if a drug is prescribed by its proprietary ('brand' or 'trade') name, then the pharmacist supplying that medication must use that brand.

In addition to the names that are commonly used in practice, other naming systems exist. For example, each drug has a chemical name: chemical names are usually derived from a formal scientific naming system, but they can be long, complex and impractical to use. Two chemical names are illustrated in Figure 4.3.

As well as chemical names, some groups of medicines are named after the chemical families to which they belong – for example, the penicillins (e.g. amoxicillin), benzodiazepines (e.g. diazepam and temazepam) and the phenothiazines (e.g. chlorpromazine and prochlorperazine), see Figure 4.4.

Internationally, a generic name, known as the 'international non-proprietary name' (INN), is issued by the World Health Organization (WHO) in several languages. In the UK, the British approved name (BAN) of a medicine is used in the BNF. The BAN is a name that is assigned to a medicine for regulatory purposes:

> *A British Approved Name (BAN) is the official non-proprietary name (also known as a generic name) given to a pharmaceutical substance for use in the UK. BANs are short, distinctive names for substances where the systematic chemical or other scientific names are too complex for convenient use.*
>
> (Source: The British Pharmacopoeia 2013, http://www.pharmacopoeia.gov.uk/publications/british-approved-names.php, accessed 6 August, 2016)

While efforts are made to co-ordinate these various standards, differences may arise. Paracetamol (INN) is called acetaminophen in the USA. Efforts continue to standardise medication names while preserving patient safety – for example, in the use of adrenaline (predominant in the UK) versus epinephrine (a term that is more universally recognised).

## Endings

In order to facilitate understanding (and pronunciation) of medication names, common endings (suffixes) can be found (Figure 4.5). Some drugs have been named historically and their use in language precedes that of the current naming systems. Therefore, while this rule can be used as a helpful hint to recognise drug names, exceptions do exist.

# 5 Numeracy and medicines management

**Figure 5.1** The seven base SI units

| Base quantity | Name | Symbol |
|---|---|---|
| **Length** | Metre | m |
| **Mass** | Kilogram | kg |
| **Time** | Second | s |
| **Electric current** | Ampere | A |
| **Thermodynamic temperature** | Kelvin | K |
| **Amount of a substance** | Mole | mol |
| **Luminous intensity** | Candela | Cd |

**Figure 5.2** The prefixes for the SI base units. The most commonly used are highlighted in yellow. The typical range of use in healthcare practice is additionally italicised

| Factor | Name | Symbol | Factor | Name | Symbol |
|---|---|---|---|---|---|
| $10^{24}$ | Yotta | Y | *$10^{-1}$* | *Deci* | *d* |
| $10^{21}$ | Zetta | Z | *$10^{-2}$* | *Centi* | *c* |
| $10^{18}$ | Exa | E | *$10^{-3}$* | *Milli* | *m* |
| $10^{15}$ | Peta | P | *$10^{-6}$* | *Micro* | *µ* |
| $10^{12}$ | Tera | T | *$10^{-9}$* | *Nano* | *n* |
| $10^{9}$ | Giga | G | $10^{-12}$ | Pico | p |
| $10^{6}$ | Mega | M | $10^{-15}$ | Femto | f |
| *$10^{3}$* | *Kilo* | *k* | $10^{-18}$ | Atto | a |
| $10^{2}$ | Hecto | h | $10^{-21}$ | Zepto | z |
| $10^{1}$ | Deka | da | $10^{-24}$ | Yocto | y |

**Figure 5.3** Illustrative examples of biological unit standards for medicinal products

| Substance | Biological equivalence |
|---|---|
| **Insulin** | 1 IU is biologically equivalent to 45.5 µg of pure crystalline insulin |
| **Vitamin A** | 1 IU is equivalent to the standarised biological activity of 0.3 µg of retinol or 0.6 µg of beta carotene |

*Medicines Management for Nurses at a Glance.* First Edition. Simon Young and Ben Pitcher. © 2016 John Wiley & Sons, Ltd. Published 2016 by John Wiley & Sons, Ltd.
www.ataglanceseries.com/nursing/medicinesmanagement

The Nursing and Midwifery Council (NMC)'s essential skills clusters (ESCs), which guide the pre-registration nursing education programmes in the UK, make particular reference to the importance of numeracy and numerical assessment. A number of the ESCs identify the need to undertake calculation to a given level of competency. This is important in managing medicines safely; drug dose calculation is an important part of the nurse's role. The ESCs highlight safe and effective calculation with regard to nutrition, fluid balance and other aspects of nursing practice. Many of the calculation assessments undertaken before the point of registration require the assessment of numeracy to a level of 100% accuracy – this pass mark is designed to reflect the importance of accurate calculation in nursing practice.

Numeracy in medicines management is deceptively complex and the consequences of dosing errors are potentially serious. The process of developing numeracy skills in nursing is so complex that dedicated learning programmes (such as safeMedicate®) have been developed to ensure that the nurse is sufficiently competent to deal with the range of dosage calculation problems encountered in practice.

## Symbols

The challenges in numeracy do not only lie in making correct calculations. Understanding the range of symbols and units of measurement used is also important – for example, when considering questions such as 'Why is the amount of digoxin in digoxin tablets measured in micrograms?' When these issues are not fully understood, errors occur and patients may be harmed. In one instance, not understanding why insulin is measured in units and not in grams or milligrams resulted in nurses administering too much insulin via a volumetric syringe, rather than an insulin syringe, thereby causing a patient's death.

Symbols are important beyond the representation of numbers in the context of numeracy. In science classes (and everyday life), symbols representing units universally define recognised quantities such as mass, length and time. These units and their associated symbols were derived to measure the quantities that define the world in which we live. Most units used globally belong to the International System of Units (universally abbreviated to SI). The system was initially conceived in the late eighteenth century and developed in an attempt to unify and rationalise systems of measurement. The SI is founded on seven SI base units for seven base quantities (Figure 5.1).

These seven units form the basic set of tools with which one can define any other scientific measurement. The SI units for length (m) and time (s) are SI defined standards and can be used to derive units of measurement such as speed (distance [m]/time [s]) and acceleration (distance [m]/time$^2$[s$^2$]). Dimensional analysis using the base units gives speed a derived SI unit of $ms^{-1}$ and acceleration a derived SI unit of $ms^{-2}$. In healthcare practice, the first three base units are important because they are used in calculations associated with medication: mass, volume and more complex calculations involving infusion rates, syringe pump measurements and rates of administration. The SI base unit of temperature (Kelvin [K]) is not used in healthcare practice but the degree Celsius scale (°c) is derived from the Kelvin. The mole is also an important unit that can be found on injectable labels and is used to define molar concentration and in biochemical concepts such as osmolarity.

In addition to the symbols derived to represent the SI units, the healthcare professional will encounter the SI unit **prefixes**. Figure 5.2 illustrates 20 key prefixes used by the SI. The prefixes represent decimal fractions and multiples of the SI unit (or derived unit) in question. The key units differ by a factor of $10^3$ (× 1000) – for example, a microgram (µg) is $10^3$ (× 1000) times smaller than a milligram (mg). In medicines dosage calculations, conversion of SI units is necessary, for example, when medicines are prescribed in micrograms and the medication is only available as a concentration in milligrams. Awareness that these conversions are necessary highlights the importance of the healthcare professional understanding the SI units and applying their knowledge as part of safe and effective medicines management practice.

In addition to the SI and derived SI units, the international unit (IU) is encountered in healthcare practice. The IU is a measurement of the amount of a substance based on its biological activity or effect. The traditional way of measuring the amount of a drug that is present in a medicinal product is by mass (e.g. mg or µg) or by the amount of molecules it contains (e.g. molar solution). Many active drugs that originate from biological sources exist in a variety of forms. For example, Vitamin D is not one unitary substance: it is the name for a group of substances. The substance we know as vitamin D is made up of compounds such as ergocalciferol, cholecalciferol and sitocalciferol. The aim in having an IU for these biological products is to be able to pharmacologically compare each form and produce a standard that produces the same **biological effect**. The World Health Organization (WHO) Committee on Biological Standardisation provides a reference preparation of given agents, sets the number of IUs contained in that preparation and then sets out a scientific test (assay) to compare other preparations with the reference preparation.

## Illustrative biological unit standards for medicinal products

If a manufacturer wishes to produce an insulin preparation for use in humans or animals, the potency of the insulin is not measured by the amount (mg or µg per insulin per mL) of the suspension but by comparing the activity of the insulin with the biological standard in Figure 5.3.

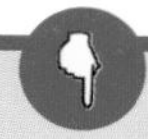

### Clinical pointers

Whilst it is scientifically accurate to use the abbreviations IU for insulin units or µg for micrograms they should not be used on medication charts or patient notes.

Due to the risk of misinterpretation, 'units' and 'micrograms' should always be written in full.

# Clinical pharmacokinetics I

**Figure 6.1** This figure integrates the four main features of pharmacokinetics (ADME) and the main routes of administration of medication. Note that the IV route bypasses absorption and the topical route is used to achieve a local effect and minimise absorption

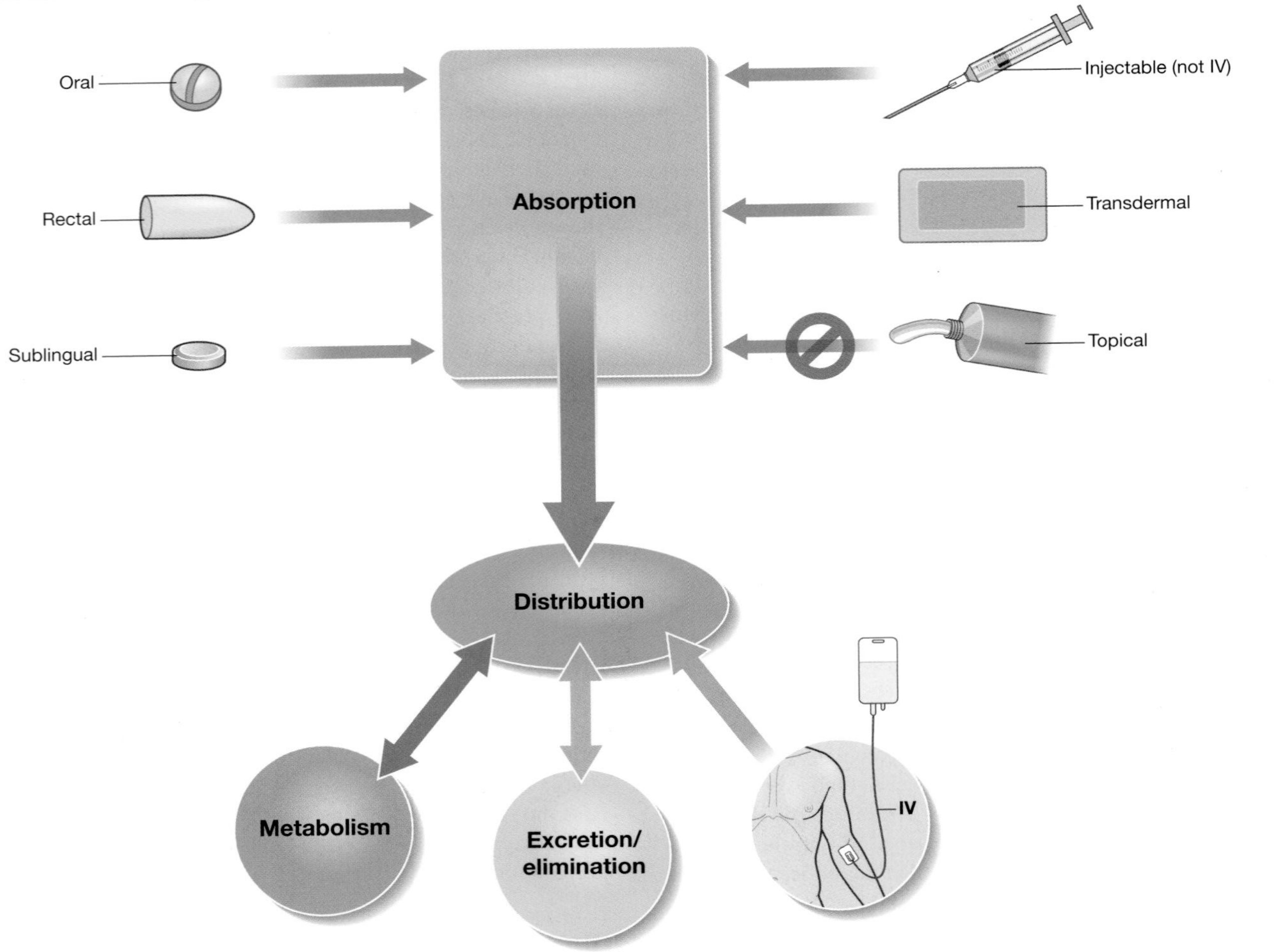

Oral
Rectal
Sublingual
Absorption
Injectable (not IV)
Transdermal
Topical
Distribution
Metabolism
Excretion/ elimination
IV

*Medicines Management for Nurses at a Glance*. First Edition. Simon Young and Ben Pitcher. © 2016 John Wiley & Sons, Ltd. Published 2016 by John Wiley & Sons, Ltd.
www.ataglanceseries.com/nursing/medicinesmanagement

Pharmacology can be broadly defined as the study of drugs and medicines. The science encompasses many aspects of the study of medicines including drug design and discovery, the sources of medicinal products, and the study of chemical structure and how that influences drug action.

Clinical pharmacology is the facet of pharmacology that considers the interaction between medicines and the human body. An understanding of the principles of clinical pharmacology is an important element of safe and effective medicines management. Clinical pharmacology will be considered in the following chapters but can be classified into the subjects of pharmacokinetics and pharmacodynamics.

Clinical pharmacokinetics describes the influence that the human body has on drugs or foreign chemicals over a given time. The science of pharmacokinetics encompasses complex mathematical modelling of the movement of a drug through the body. When considering pharmacokinetics in the context of medicines management, a more anatomical and less mathematical appreciation of pharmacokinetics can be made. The pharmacokinetics of a particular drug agent is best studied by considering four processes, known by the acronym ADME (Figure 6.1):

- Absorption (A).
- Distribution (D).
- Metabolism (M).
- Excretion (E).

## Absorption

Absorption describes the process of the drug agent moving from its site of administration into the general circulation. Most drugs are administered via a licensed route (the route of administration tested and recommended by the manufacturer) and designed to enter the general circulation. From the general circulation, a drug may then have access to the site of action (the part of the body it is designed to treat). Some drugs exert their action where applied – for example, many creams and drugs such as vancomycin (an antibiotic designed to treat infections of the gastro-intestinal tract).

Drug entities must cross various barriers to get to the general circulation. Many drugs move by passive diffusion (i.e. movement from an area of high concentration to one of low concentration). To be absorbed after it has been swallowed, a drug must move from the small intestine, through the gut wall, through a blood vessel wall into the hepato-portal circulation, through the liver and eventually into the systemic circulation. Some drugs use active transport mechanisms (similar to 'pumps') to facilitate their movement across the cell membrane. Other drugs use both passive diffusion and active transport mechanisms, depending on factors such as their concentration in the gut (e.g. vitamin $B_1$).

Many factors can influence the absorption of medication from the gut. The presence of food and fluid in the stomach or combinations of drugs given together, such as indigestion remedies, can have an impact on absorption. Many other factors may influence the absorption of drugs administered by other routes. A failure to appreciate these factors may influence the desired therapeutic outcome.

Rates of absorption from patches and slow- or modified-release capsules are important considerations in medicines management. Intravenous (IV) drugs are the only group of drugs that do not undergo absorption. IV administration results in 100% of the drug getting into the circulation by bypassing the need for the drug to be absorbed, while other routes may only allow a fraction of the administered drug to reach the blood. This concept is described by the phrase **bioavailability**, which refers to the proportion of administered drug that reaches the general circulation.

## Distribution

When a drug has been absorbed or introduced directly into the blood stream, it frequently needs to be transported to the site of action (distribution). Most modern drug agents are not 'magic bullets' and will travel indiscriminately in the circulation, reaching not only the site of action but all parts of the body. This indiscriminate behaviour of drugs leads to the most common side effects experienced by patients when using pharmacologically active agents.

Blood flow is an important factor in determining the exact distribution of a drug agent. Organs that are well perfused (e.g. the kidneys and heart) will generally receive a plentiful supply of most drug agents. Tissues such as fat and bone, which are poorly perfused, will receive less drug in a given time and it may take longer for the drug to reach an adequate concentration for therapeutic effect on those tissues.

### Barriers to distribution

The human body possesses natural structures that protect vital organs from the harmful influences of drugs. The brain, for obvious reasons, must be protected from drugs and other potentially toxic chemicals. The circulation of the brain possesses specific cellular formations (the **blood–brain barrier**) that prevent the passage of many chemicals from the general circulation to the brain. This protective mechanism is useful for survival, but a hindrance to pharmacological therapy. To exert their actions, all drugs that act on the central nervous system (CNS) must pass through the blood–brain barrier in adequate concentration. The placental barrier serves a similar purpose in protecting the developing foetus.

### Protein binding

For drugs to cross from the circulation into organs and tissues, they must be dissolved in tissue fluids or plasma. In pharmacokinetic terms, a drug that is dissolved in plasma and able to diffuse into tissues is called a **free drug**. Some drugs will bind to the protein components of plasma (e.g. albumin or $\alpha_1$-acid glycoprotein) and become a **bound drug**. A drug that is bound to plasma protein is unable to diffuse from the circulation into tissues and exert its action. A delicate balance is set up between the amount of drug that is free and that which is bound. The dose of drug that should be administered takes account of this binding and is part of the consideration taken to achieve the desired plasma concentration. Errors in medication administration can affect this delicate balance and result in issues such as increased prevalence of side effects and toxicity.

# Clinical pharmacokinetics II

**Figure 7.1** This figure illustrates the four main features of pharmacokinetics (ADME) and the main anatomical structures/physiological systems that are responsible for executing those processes. Note that the two-way arrows illustrate that in reality the ADME processes cycle continuously rather than as a linear process

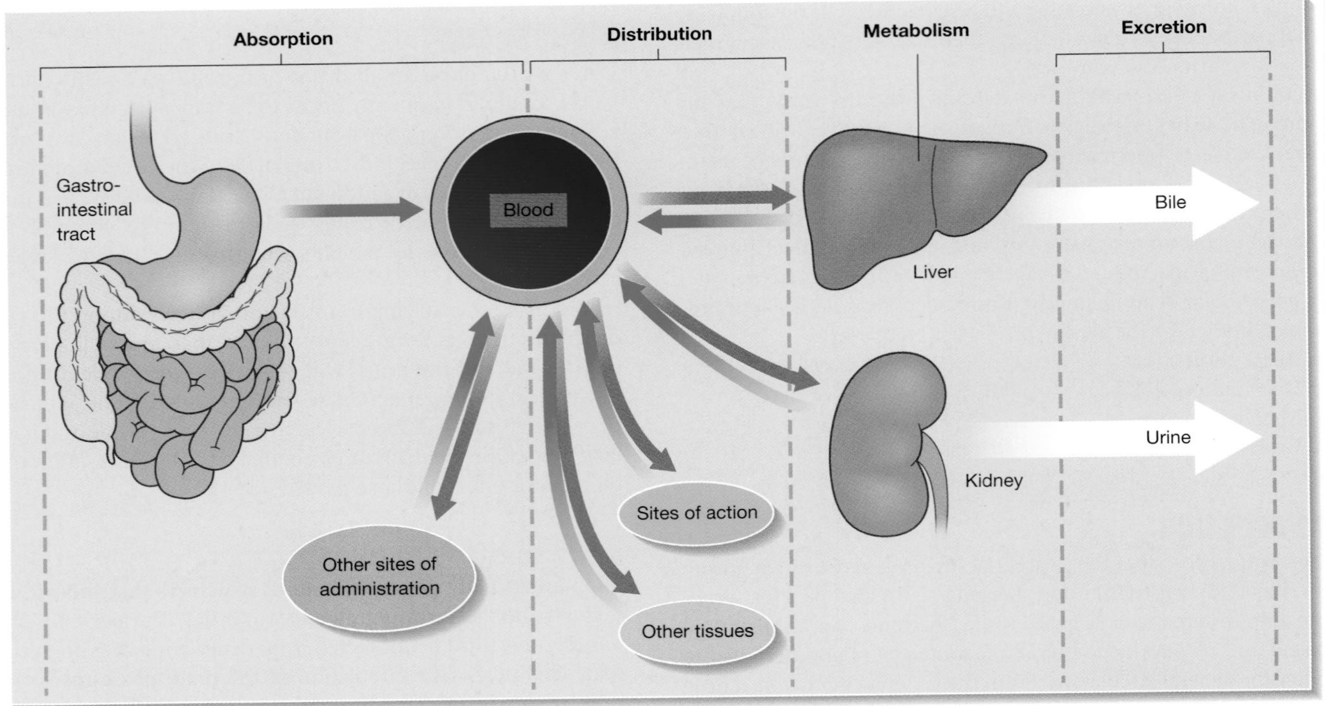

Clinical pharmacokinetics can be considered as four processes: absorption, distribution, metabolism and excretion (Figure 7.1). Absorption and distribution are discussed in detail in Chapter 6. This chapter will explore metabolism and excretion.

## Metabolism

If the human body did not possess the capacity to metabolise and excrete drugs, they would never leave the body after their administration. The drug would continually circulate in the blood stream exerting its effect. For example, a hypnotic such as temazepam that was neither metabolised nor excreted would continually circulate around the body unchanged and continuously exerting its effect, keeping you asleep forever!

The body possesses efficient systems for biotransformation (metabolism) that serve many purposes. The most important aim of drug metabolism is to modify chemicals with the primary aim of making them more water soluble and more easily excreted. The dosing regime of a drug is designed so that the amount of drug administered is balanced against the rates of metabolism and excretion in order to maintain an appropriate plasma concentration. When considering initiating drug therapy, liver (hepatic) function and the way the drug is metabolised becomes an important consideration especially if there is hepatic impairment (Chapter 46).

There are enzymes (Chapter 11) present in the liver that are responsible for undertaking drug metabolism. While there are other tissues and organs where drug metabolism takes place, such as the kidneys and plasma, the liver is the primary organ involved.

In classifying drug metabolism pharmacokinetically, it can be divided into two phases.

### Phase I

The reactions catalysed in phase I of metabolism are simple chemical changes that are made to the drug such as oxidation, reduction and/or hydrolysis. The most common group of enzymes considered when studying phase I metabolism is the cytochrome P450 isoenzyme family (CYP450). The primary aim of this phase is to make the drugs pharmacologically inactive and more water soluble, and to prepare the metabolite for phase II.

### Phase II

If the metabolites of phase I are not sufficiently hydrophilic (water soluble), then phase II serves to conjugate (add) endogenous chemicals to the structure to enhance the drug's water solubility. Endogenous chemicals involved include glucuronates and sulphates. These more water-soluble compounds are more easily excreted by the kidneys.

Certain drugs only undergo phase I metabolism, others only phase II metabolism and some drugs undergo very little or no metabolism at all. Some drugs undergo phase II metabolism and then phase I. Certain drugs – for example, levodopa (used to treat Parkinson's disease) – are inactive in the body until some biotransformation takes place. These drugs are known as pro-drugs. Certain drugs (e.g. the antidepressant fluoxetine) are transformed into metabolites that are also active, and these metabolites are partially responsible for the therapeutic activity of the drug agent.

## Excretion

### Renal excretion

Most drugs are excreted by the kidneys. In initiating drug therapy, the patient's renal function is considered. Any changes in renal function often require adjustment of the dosage or dosage frequency of a drug in order to avoid its accumulating in the body. Such accumulation may result in increased side effects and eventually toxicity (poisoning).

The body has the capacity to excrete drugs through any path by which water leaves the body (e.g. they are excreted in faeces, tears, breast milk, sweat and even water vapour that is exhaled in breathing).

Drug agents are either excreted after metabolic processes or unchanged. To understand the process of renal excretion of drugs, it is necessary to understand the physiology of the kidney and how the kidneys filter plasma. However, some basic principles apply. Very water-soluble, unbound drugs will freely diffuse from the blood stream into the glomerulus of the kidney and be excreted. Drugs bound to plasma proteins will not pass from the blood stream. More lipophilic drugs tend to get resorbed into the blood stream after initial excretion. Certain drugs that have specific physico-chemical properties will be actively secreted by the kidneys.

The kidneys are by far the most efficient mechanism by which drugs leave the body, and an understanding of the principles of renal function and its measurement are important for a full understanding of the process of excretion. When a patient has impaired renal function, some important patient and drug characteristics must be considered before prescribing decisions are made. These considerations have a bearing on those healthcare professionals who are responsible for taking decisions with regard to the administration of drugs in practice. Declining renal function is associated with aging, and renal function in children is different from that in adults. This accounts for some of the reasons for adjusting doses in geriatric and paediatric practice.

### Enterohepatic recycling

Some drugs are excreted (and concentrated) into bile. The drug is then excreted into the intestine where a process of resorption may take place. This process is known as enterohepatic recycling or circulation. It is believed to be important in oral contraceptive pill failure when broad-spectrum antibiotics are taken. It may also play a role in oral contraceptive failure associated with diarrhoea.

Pharmacokinetic knowledge in its entirety helps us understand many aspects of managing medicines in health care, including starting dose, reasons for dose adjustment and how long it takes drugs to 'start working'.

# 8 Routes of administration I

Figure 8.1 This figure illustrates how the three most common injectable routes of administration deliver the drug through the skin into three distinct depths and tissue types

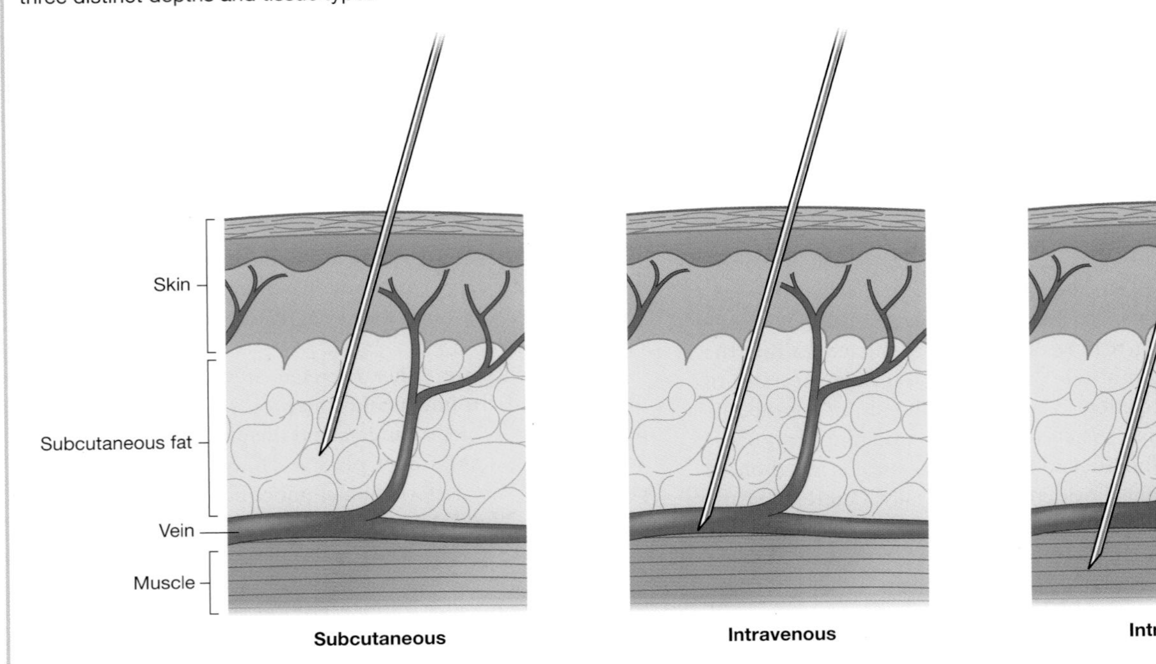


There are a variety of ways that a drug can get into the body (Figure 8.1). These are called routes of administration. It is important to understand why different drugs are administered via different routes. Each route has advantages and disadvantages. If all routes of administration were equally effective, we would take all our drugs in tablet form.

## Oral

The most common means of administering medication is orally with tablets and liquids, swallowing the drug in the same way as we would food. This uses the machinery of the body, which is intended to take things from the outside world (sugar, fat, water) and internalise them. Because of this, the oral route is the most common route that we use, and in most cases we only use alternative routes if we have to.

### Advantages

- **Low cost**
  Oral preparations are relatively inexpensive to manufacture. This often makes them the cheapest way to provide medication.
- **Easy**
  Most people find swallowing medication easy, or at least easier than injecting it. It requires no special training and is generally associated with no extra risk.
- **Versatile**
  Oral preparations are available in different forms (tablets, syrups, etc.) that allow them to be tailored to different clinical circumstances. They can also be prepared in slow-release formulations that allow a single dose of drug to be effective over a long period of time.

### Disadvantages

- **The destructive nature of the GI tract**
  The digestive system is designed to break down foods into simpler molecules. Drugs that are swallowed will suffer the same fate. If a drug is totally destroyed by the digestive system, then the oral route cannot be used. This is why insulin must be administered via injection and cannot be taken orally.
- **Food**
  Things that you eat can affect how a drug is absorbed. This can require drugs to be taken at specific times in relation to when you have eaten.
- **First-pass metabolism**
  Everything that is absorbed from the intestines travels to the liver. The liver is the prime site of metabolism. This can result in large amounts of a drug being metabolised before it reaches its intended site of action. This can make the oral route very inefficient.

## Intravenous

This is the administration of a drug directly into the blood supply either through a needle or, more usually, a cannula. The intravenous (IV) route is used when we need to get something into the blood quickly or when other routes are not possible. The most common drugs that are given intravenously are antibiotics, strong painkillers or replacement fluids. While the term 'IV' could refer to the administration of a drug into any vein, it is usually into a larger peripheral vein in the arm or wrist.

### Advantages

- **Fast acting**
  Reaches the blood supply very quickly, making it good in emergencies or where the dose needs to be titrated carefully.
- **Bypasses first-pass metabolism**
  This route gets the drug directly into the blood stream, bypassing the digestive system and the liver, and is therefore more efficient than the oral route.

### Disadvantages

- **Training required**
  It can be difficult to locate a vein or secure access, and failing to administer the drug directly into the vein can cause considerable harm to the surrounding tissues.
- **High cost**
  IV products are expensive to manufacture because they need to be sterile. They also require sterile equipment (syringes, needles, giving sets, etc.) for their use.
- **Access**
  For the drug to be administered, the needle or catheter must be successfully inserted into a vein. This can be difficult when the patient is unwell.
- **Risk of toxicity**
  The rapidity of this route can be a pitfall. Because the full dose of a drug can reach the blood very quickly, there is an increased risk of accidental overdose.
- **Risk of infection**
  Bypassing the natural barrier of infection of the skin carries an extra infection risk.

## Intramuscular

Rather than injecting into the vein, the drug is injected into the muscle. A smaller range of drugs are given by this route. Examples include immunisations and antipsychotics.

### Advantages

- **Depot injections**
  The muscle can tolerate a volume of drug of a reasonable size. This can be used to create a reservoir of drug within the muscle, which will slowly absorb over time, creating a longer-lasting effect.
- Bypasses first-pass metabolism

### Disadvantages

- **Training required**
  The needle must only be inserted into specific areas of muscle to ensure that the drug is not accidentally injected into a vein or at risk of damaging a nerve.
- **Unpredictable rate of absorption**
  The rate at which the drug is absorbed can vary depending on the use of the muscle.

## Subcutaneous

The drug is injected into the subcutaneous fat layer that lies underneath the skin and above the muscle. This is a relatively simple method of administering drugs that cannot be administered orally.

This is most commonly seen as the method of administering insulin to diabetics.

### Advantages

- Bypasses first-pass metabolism
- **Can be self-administered**
  Requires little training and therefore patients can easily be taught to administer the drug themselves.
- **Predictable rate of absorption**
  Can be used for drugs that require very specific dosing (such as insulin).

### Disadvantages

- **Discomfort**
  Repeated injections can cause pain at the site.
- **Local effects**
  The site of injection can be affected by the administered drug, even if it is intended to act systemically (e.g. localised bruising around the injection site of anticoagulants).

# 9 Routes of administration II

**Figure 9.1** Diagram illustrating how a transdermal patch works

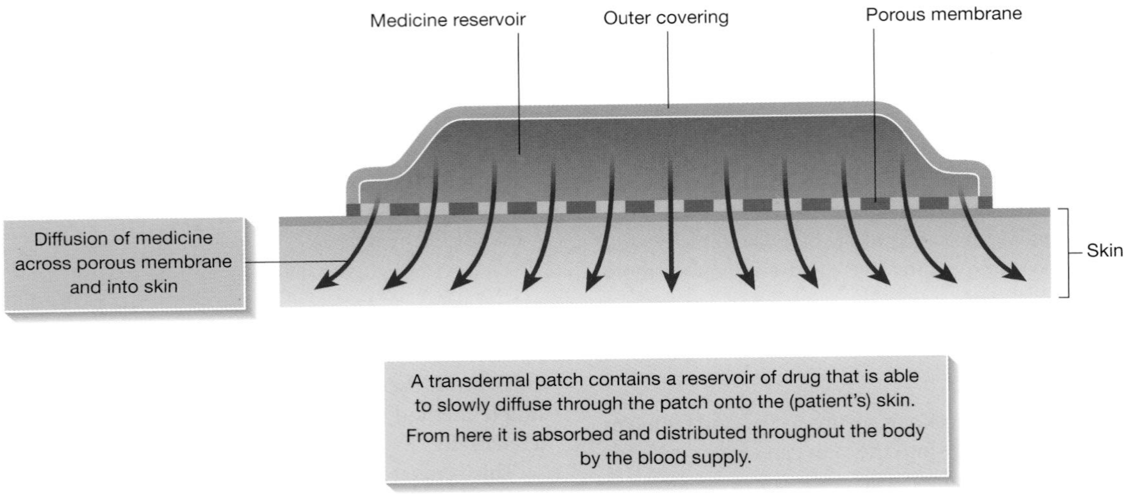

**Figure 9.2** Suggested sites for the positioning of a transdermal patch

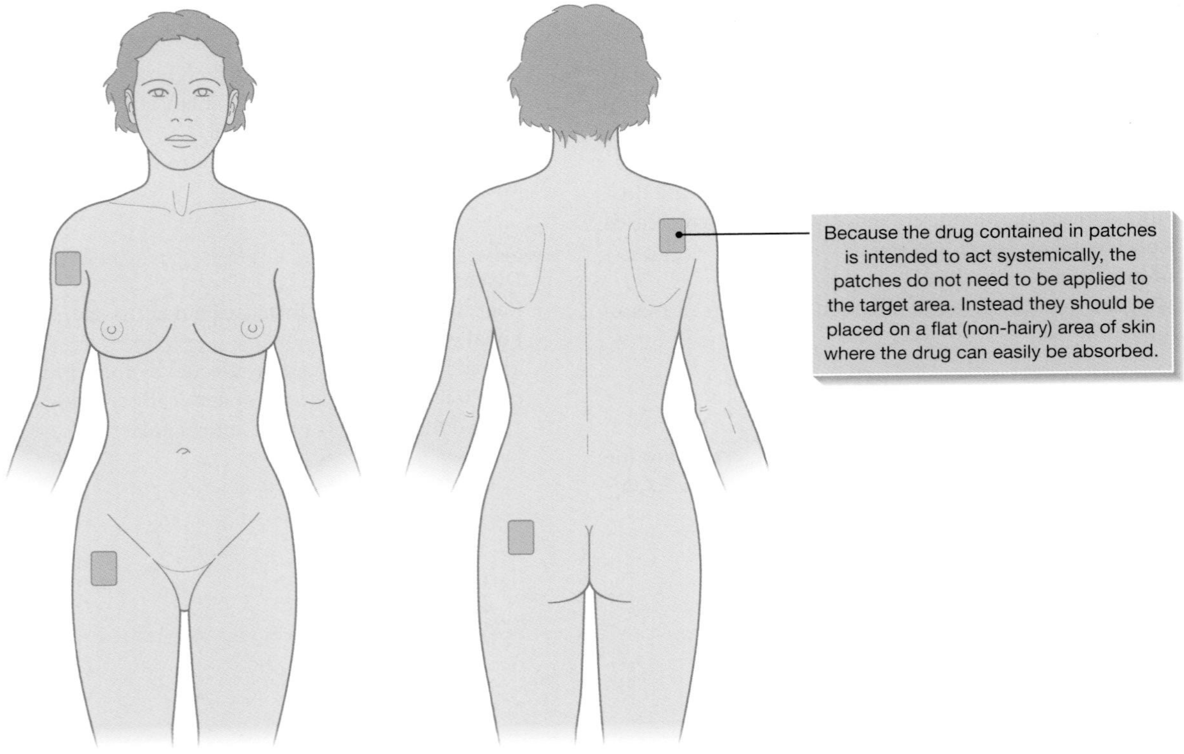

While the oral or injectable routes are the most frequently used in clinical practice, there are other routes of administration that may be more beneficial to patients. These routes can help us overcome certain problems but they have their own distinct drawbacks (Figure 9.1).

## Inhaled

Inhaling a drug directly into the lungs can be a very effective way of delivering a drug to the tissues of the lung. This is useful in treating respiratory diseases such as asthma or chronic

*Medicines Management for Nurses at a Glance*. First Edition. Simon Young and Ben Pitcher. © 2016 John Wiley & Sons, Ltd. Published 2016 by John Wiley & Sons, Ltd.
www.ataglanceseries.com/nursing/medicinesmanagement

obstructive pulmonary disease (COPD). It can also be a way of rapidly delivering drugs into the blood stream for a systemic effect like anaesthesia.

### Advantages

- **Rapid**
  Can be used to deliver a drug to the lungs quickly to provide fast relief of symptoms.

### Disadvantages

- **Inhaler technique**
  If a patient is unable to use an inhaler correctly, they may not receive the full dose and therefore may not receive the full benefit of the drug, leading to a worsening of their condition and an increased risk of hospitalisation.
  Patients using aerosol inhalers (known as metered-dose-inhalers or MDIs) will usually get the best results using a spacer.

## Topical

Drugs that are administered directly to the skin or external mucous membranes are said to be 'topical'. These can include creams, ointments and eye drops. Topical drugs are primarily intended to act on the surface of the body, directly affecting the skin; however, this is not always the case. Some topical agents (such as ibuprofen gel) cross the skin to affect the tissue beneath (see Chapters 41 and 42 for more detail on skin treatments).

### Advantages

- **Local effect with reduced systemic effect or side effect**
  The topical route is useful because it allows you to apply drugs directly to the affected area without the drug having to be circulated through the whole body via the blood stream. This can avoid any side effects or even the potential toxicity of the drug. For example, ibuprofen can be administered topically onto a sore ankle with lower risk of the gastric irritation that can occur when it is administered orally.

### Disadvantages

- **Difficult to regulate dosage**
  Because the topical administration of a drug involves creams squeezed out onto the finger and then rubbed onto the skin, or fluid dripped into the eyes (most of which will immediately run out), it can be hard to know exactly how much is given to a patient.

## Transdermal

Drugs can be administered via patches. These patches contain a reservoir of a drug that slowly seeps out and passes through the skin into the body. Examples of transdermal patches include analgesics, nicotine patches and hormone replacement therapy.

### Advantages

- **Easy to administer**
  Can be self-administered with minimal training.
- **Predictable rate of absorption**
  The rate at which the drug seeps out of the patch and enters the body is very consistent.

### Disadvantages

- **Slow onset of action**
  It takes time for the drug to seep through the skin. This means that there can be a notable delay between the application of the patch and its taking effect. This is particularly important when applying an analgesic patch.
- **Can be indiscreet**
  The patches that are often applied to the upper arm are visible (although other areas of the body can be used, see Figure 9.2). Some patients can find this embarrassing.
- **Effect of heat on absorption**
  Exposing the patch to heat can affect its functioning.

## Sublingual

Some drugs can be administered by being placed in the mouth, underneath the tongue. Although this route involves placing drugs into the mouth, we consider it distinct from the oral route because the drug is not swallowed. This route is commonly used to deliver anti-anginal medication such as glyceryl tri-nitrate (GTN).

### Advantages

- **Bypasses first-pass metabolism**
  This route bypasses the liver and is therefore more efficient than the oral route.
- **Fast acting**
  Drugs administered by this route get into the blood stream quickly and start to work almost immediately. This is very useful in urgent situations such as need for relief from angina.

### Disadvantages

- **Dose restriction**
  There is a limit to how much of a drug can be kept in the mouth without either spitting it out or swallowing it, resulting in the patient receiving less of the intended dose.

## Rectal

Some drugs can be administered by placing them in the rectum as a suppository or enema. This route is commonly used to administer analgesics in suppository form, anticonvulsants when a patient is having an epileptic seizure and laxatives to relieve severe constipation.

### Advantages

- **Bypasses first-pass metabolism**
- **Accessibility**
  This route can provide an opportunity to administer drugs if other routes (such as oral) are unavailable.

### Disadvantages

- **Inconsistent rate of absorption**
  This makes it hard to know how much drug a patient has received and how quickly it will take effect. This problem can be compounded by the potential for suppositories to pass out of the body before the drug has been absorbed.
- **Can be viewed as distasteful**
  Many people find the prospect of receiving a drug rectally as embarrassing or distressing. This can lead patients to refuse this potentially beneficial route.

There are a variety of routes of administration that allow drugs to be delivered to the site of action. Each route has its advantages and disadvantages. Understanding this can help us select the most appropriate route for any given clinical situation.

# 10 Pharmacodynamics I

**Figure 10.1** A simple membrane-spanning protein

Binding site (receptor)
Outside the cell
A membrane-spanning protein comprised of amino acids
Cell membrane
Inside the cell

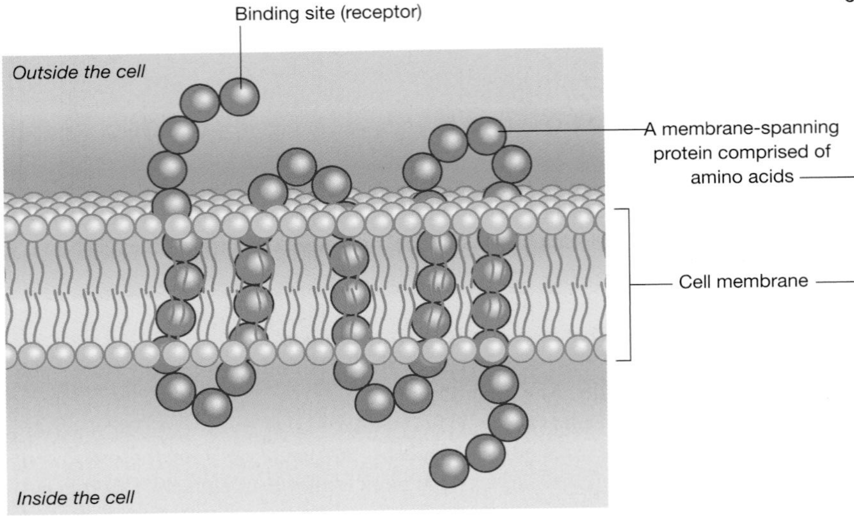

**Figure 10.2** A diagrammatic representation of a membrane-spanning protein

Binding site (receptor)

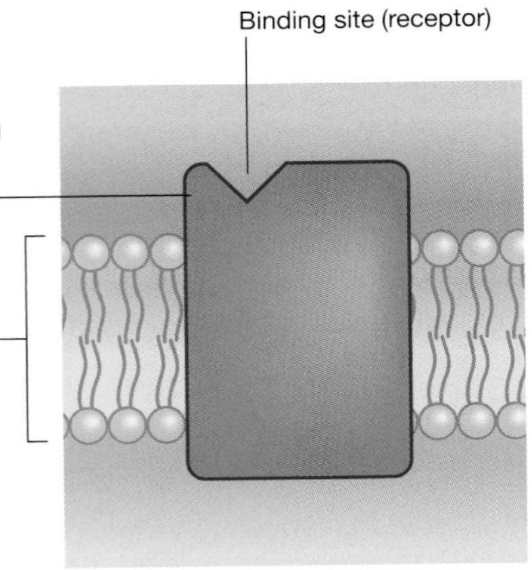

**Figure 10.3** A second messenger system

Receptor
G-protein
Enzyme

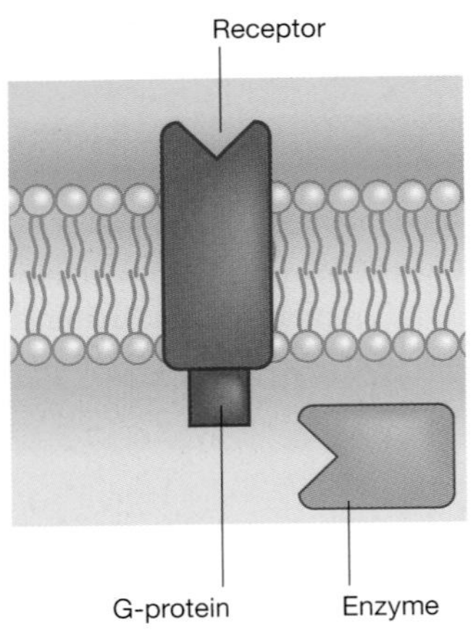

**Figure 10.4** The step-by-step process of a second messenger system

1. An agonist binds to the receptor, found on the external portion of a membrane-spanning protein
Agonist
G-protein
This causes a conformational change in the membrane-spanning protein
2. The conformational change causes the G-protein to be released into the cytosol
The G-protein can then bind to enzymes within the cell
3. When the G-protein binds to the enzyme it activates. This will facilitate some form of metabolic process within the cell

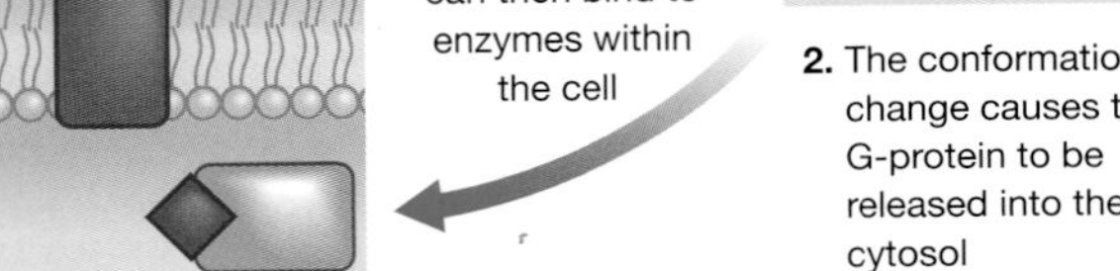

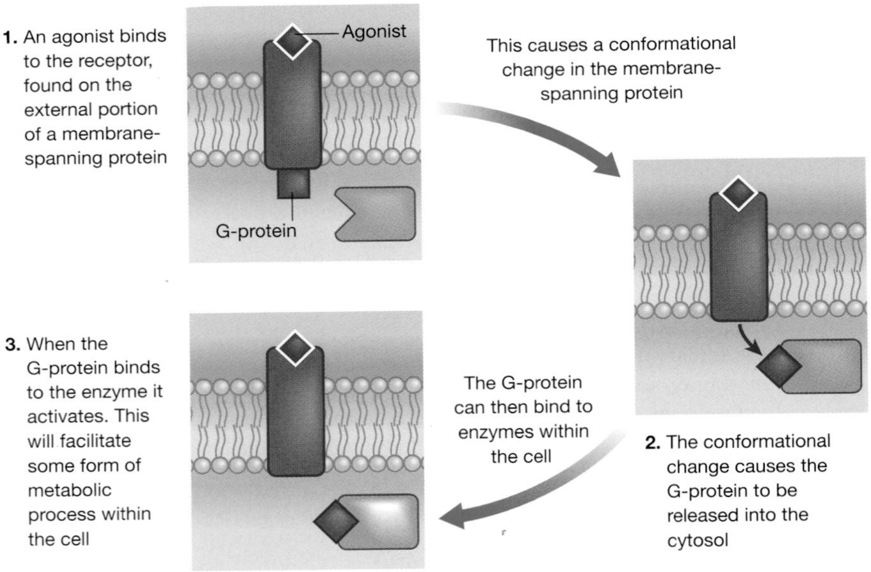

**Figure 10.5** Step-by-step receptor-mediated ion channel

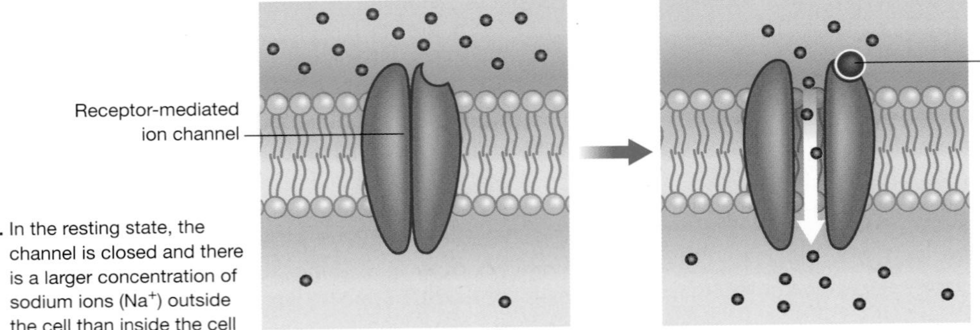

Receptor-mediated ion channel
1. In the resting state, the channel is closed and there is a larger concentration of sodium ions ($Na^+$) outside the cell than inside the cell
Agonist
2. When an agonist binds to the receptor it causes a conformational change in the membrane-spanning protein. This change opens the channel and allows the ions to flow along the concentration gradient, from where they are in high concentration to where they are in low concentration

## What is pharmacodynamics?

While **pharmacokinetics** looks at what the body does to the drug, **pharmacodynamics** looks at what the drug does to the body – specifically, how the drug molecules interact within the body, what they interact with, and how they cause their effects.

The aspects of pharmacodynamics can be expressed as the:
- biochemical and physiological effects of drugs on the body or on micro-organisms or parasites within or on the body
- mechanisms of drug action
- relationship between drug concentration and effect.

## Why do chemicals have such varied but specific effects on the body?

This is an important issue to get to grips with. Why does introducing a specific chemical to the body produce such a specific and strong response in the body? The answer helps explain the way that most drugs work. A large number of drugs work by stimulating or blocking the body's own control mechanisms.

The body has a variety of systems and processes in place that allow it to control its internal environment. This can involve the use of the endocrine system (i.e. hormones) or the autonomic nervous system (i.e. neurotransmitters). Both hormones and neurotransmitters are chemicals that bind to **receptors**, which are proteins found on the surface of specific cells, causing a response within the cell or associated organ. A drug can mimic the neurotransmitter or hormone binding to the receptor and either stimulate or block its action.

Other biochemical processes are regulated by **enzymes**, specialist proteins that allow specific chemical reactions to occur. Drugs that stimulate, inhibit or destroy these enzymes will dramatically affect these processes.

## Receptors

A receptor is a binding site with which a chemical (known as an **agonist**) can interact, effecting some sort of change. In the body the chemical might be a hormone or neurotransmitter. A lot of drugs mimic these endogenous (produced within the body) chemicals, allowing us to hijack or block the body's own control mechanisms.

The receptor is often part of, or connected to, some form of protein. These proteins are long chains of amino acids, partly outside a cell and partly inside it. These are called membrane-spanning proteins (Figure 10.1). When a chemical binds to the portion of the protein on the outside of the cell, it causes the protein to change shape. This may activate some form of cellular process or it might create an opening that will allow ions (e.g. $Na^+$ or $K^+$) to pass into or out of the cell.

In reality, the proteins involved can be far longer and far more complicated. These proteins are presented diagrammatically as simpler shapes (Figure 10.2).

## Second messenger systems

As mentioned earlier, when an agonist binds to a receptor it produces a response within the cell. This is often achieved by the use of a **second messenger**. We have already established that the receptors are usually part of a membrane-spanning protein. In these systems, there is a separate G-protein attached to the interior portion of the membrane-spanning protein: this is the second messenger (Figure 10.3). When an agonist (which is the **first messenger**) successfully binds to the external part of the receptor, it causes a conformational change. This makes the second messenger protein break away from the membrane-spanning protein. The second messenger protein then binds to and activates enzymes within the cytosol, essentially 'switching on' some form of reaction within the cell (Figure 10.4).

This system is used throughout the body. For example, the receptors that respond to adrenaline use second messenger systems.

## Ion channels

So far we have looked at receptors that, when bound to by an agonist, activate something within the cell. Another type of receptor is one that is attached to an ion channel (Figure 10.5).

Ion channels are a collection of membrane-spanning proteins that are grouped together to form a channel. These channels can be opened or closed allowing (or preventing if closed) the movement of ions from one side of the cell membrane to the other.

The movement of ions across the membrane is essential for the activity of cells. This is particularly true in excitable cells such as nerve cells or the cells of the heart, where the movement of ions facilitates nerve impulses and the contraction of the heart muscle. Many of these channels are opened in response to an agonist binding to a receptor. When the agonist binds to the receptor, it causes a conformational change in the membrane-spanning protein that opens a passage through the centre of the channel, allowing ions to pass through. In the body this agonist might be a neurotransmitter or a hormone.

Many drugs bind to these receptors, allowing us to control the opening and closing of channels and the activity of the cells and tissues they are attached to.

# 11 Pharmacodynamics II

Figure 11.1 An agonist is any chemical that binds to a receptor and elicits a positive response from the adjoining cell

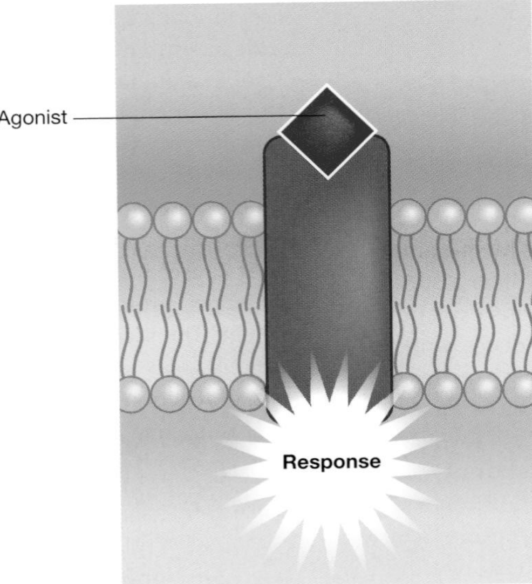


Figure 11.2 An antagonist is any chemical that binds to a receptor but elicits no response and prevents a response from occurring

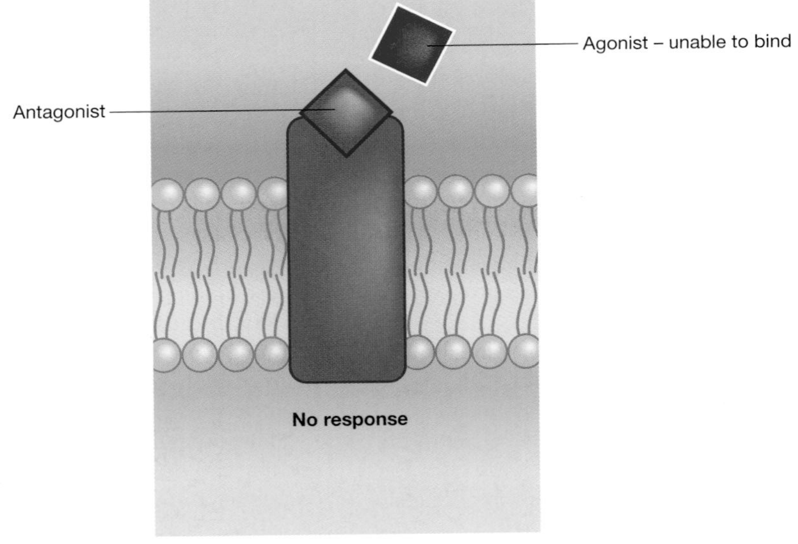

In Chapter 10 we looked at the nature of receptors and how, when they are stimulated, they can bring about changes within a cell (e.g. by opening channels or activating an enzyme). In this chapter, we will look at the chemicals that stimulate the receptors, whether they are the neurotransmitters and hormones produced naturally within the body, or whether they are introduced to the body in the form of drugs.

## Agonists and antagonists

We have discussed how chemicals can bind to receptors. In the body these chemicals are hormones and neurotransmitters. When these chemicals bind to a receptor, they effect some form of change or initiate some sort of activity.

Any chemical that binds to a receptor and elicits a positive response from the adjoining cell is known as an **agonist** (Figure 11.1). The neurotransmitter or hormone that is produced by the body and would normally stimulate the receptor is referred to as an **endogenous agonist**.

There are also chemicals that can bind to a receptor but illicit no response and in fact prevent a response from occurring. These are known as **antagonists** (Figure 11.2).

We often think of these chemicals as being either 'agonist' or 'antagonist' because they either cause a response or no response. However, this is an over-simplification. Different chemicals can illicit different degrees of response, which we benchmark against the endogenous agonist. If a chemical binds to a receptor and produces a response that is smaller than that caused by the endogenous agonist, we refer to it as a **partial agonist**. If a partial agonist is introduced to tissue where receptors are unbound by any agonists, it will bind to the receptors and create a small response. Because this small response is greater than no response, its effect will be like that of an agonist. If a partial agonist is introduced to tissue that is heavily stimulated by the endogenous agonist, it will compete for the same receptor and prevent the endogenous agonist from binding, thereby acting like an antagonist. Even though the partial agonist causes a response, it is a smaller response than that from the endogenous agonist, so the tissue is less stimulated. This can be useful in situations where a full antagonist is too 'strong'.

If an agonist causes a greater response than the endogenous agonist, it can be referred to as a **superagonist**. These can be useful when we want to stimulate a control system within the body and increase the response above what the body would normally do. An example of this can be seen with opioid analgesics. Endogenous opioids modulate the pain response and reduce the sensation of pain. Fentanyl illicits a far higher response than endogenous opioids, allowing the analgesic effect to be elevated beyond what our body can achieve on its own.

## Receptor specificity

There are different types of receptor for different types of endogenous agonist. There are receptors that respond to adrenaline (adrenergic receptors) and receptors that respond to acetylcholine (cholinergic receptors). However, there are also subtypes of receptor for each endogenous agonist found in different tissues throughout the body. They are all stimulated by the same endogenous agonist but they are all different, often precipitating different actions within the cells they are attached to. This can help explain the diverse range of actions a hormone can have: for example, how adrenaline causes smooth muscle relaxation in the bronchioles and smooth muscle constriction in the peripheral vasculature. These differences in receptor subtype provide us with therapeutic options. If we can develop a chemical that acts specifically on one subtype of receptor but not on another, we can focus the action of a drug onto one tissue type and avoid unwanted side effects caused by stimulating others. An ideal drug would be completely selective and therefore only affect the intended receptor subtype. However, ideal drugs rarely exist and most drugs that target a specific receptor subtype will still have some effect on others.

## Enzymes

In Chapter 7 we looked at enzymes as agents responsible for the metabolism of drugs. In drug metabolism, the enzymes are responsible for making changes to a drug molecule, making it inactive or easier to eliminate. However, enzymes are specialist proteins that allow specific chemical reactions to occur.

Enzymes facilitate crucial chemical reactions within the body. If enzymes are inhibited, then their associated reactions will be greatly reduced or even stop. This means that if there is some physiological process that is causing a problem, then inhibiting one of the enzymes that facilitate this process can relieve that problem. For example, the cyclooxygenase enzyme is responsible for producing inflammatory mediators that cause pain and swelling in response to injury. Anti-inflammatory drugs (such as ibuprofen) inhibit the cyclooxygenase enzyme, preventing the production of the inflammatory mediators and reducing the pain and swelling.

A large number of drugs act by inhibiting enzymes. Common examples are:

- aspirin
- ibuprofen
- statins (cholesterol-lowering drugs)
- some antihypertensives (angiotensin converting enzyme [ACE] inhibitors)
- some antidepressants (monoamine oxidase inhibitors [MAOIs]).

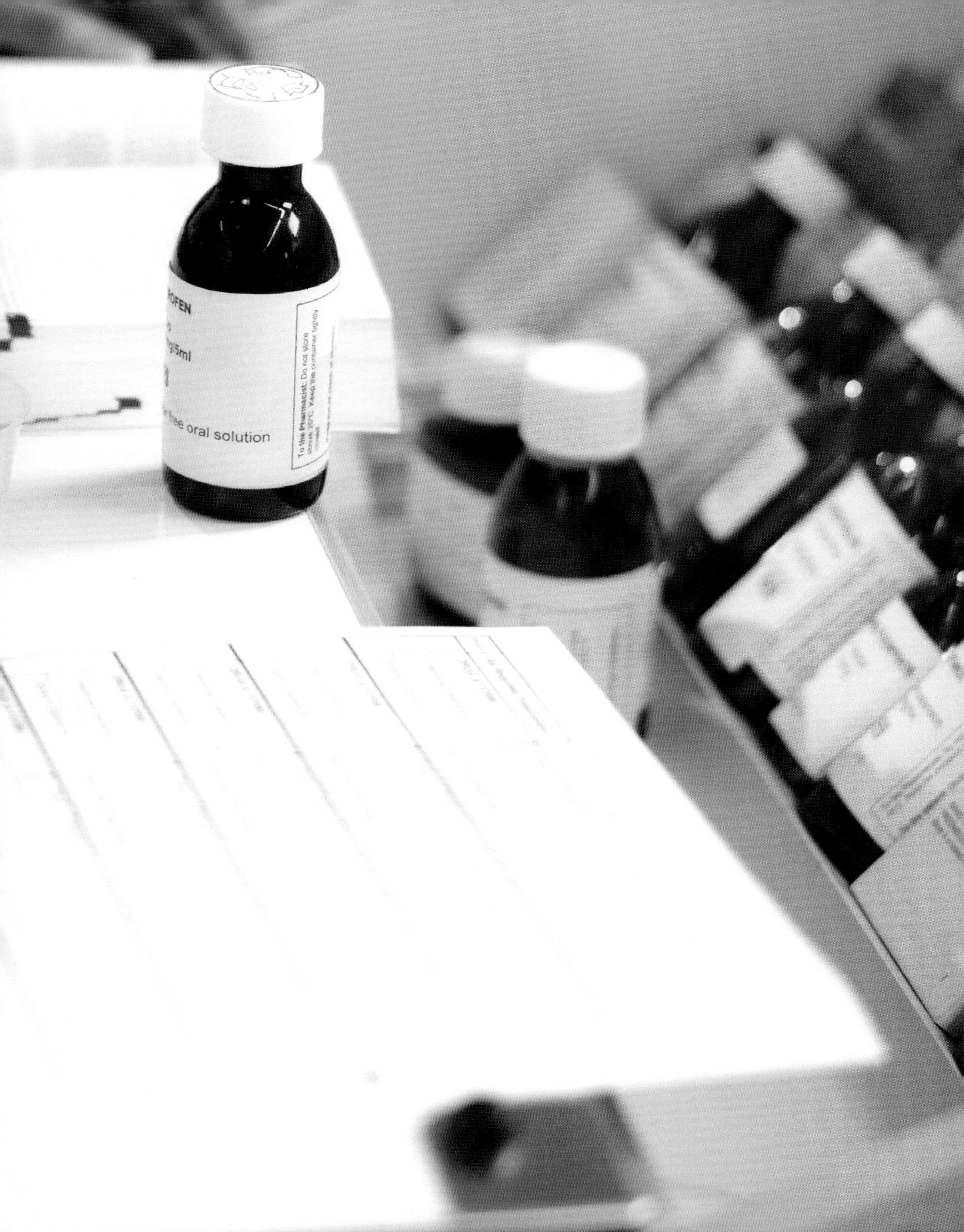
free oral solution
To the Pharmacist: Do not store
above 25°C. Keep the container tightly
closed.

# Managing medicines

## Chapters

# 12 Dyspepsia

Figure 12.1 An entry from an in-patient medication chart illustrating the key features to be considered when managing PPIs

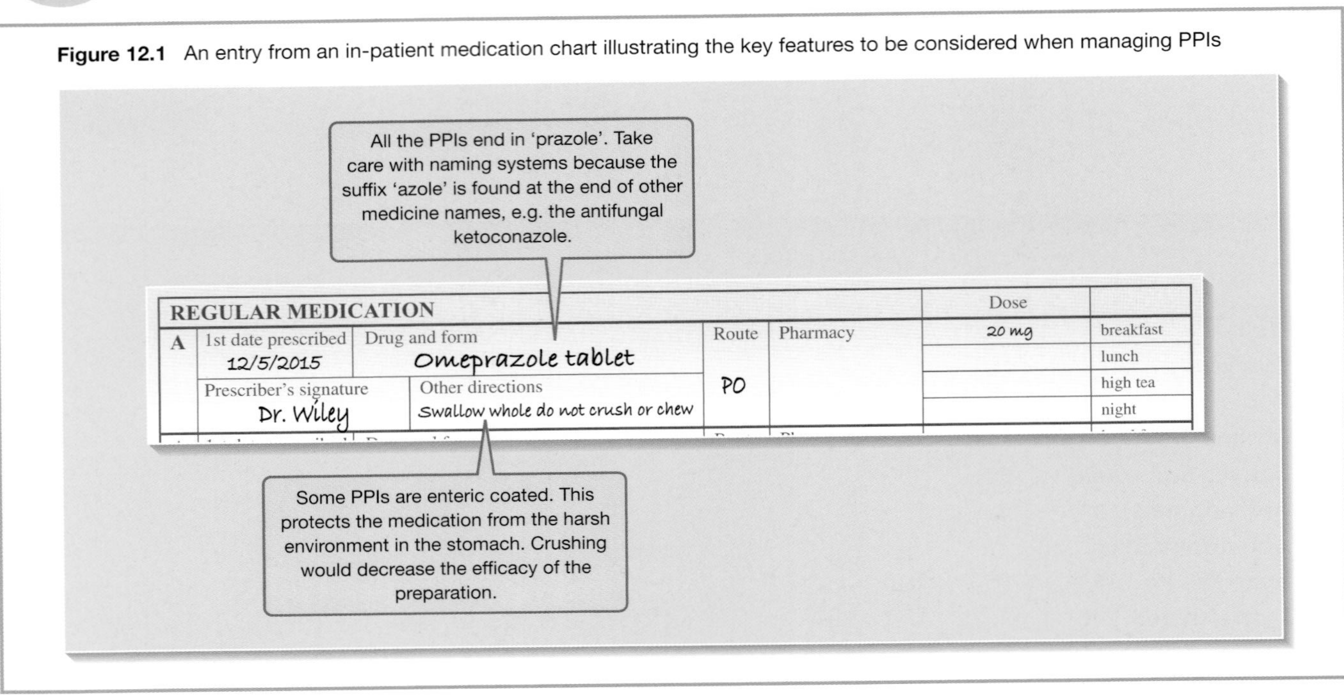


## Dyspepsia

Dyspepsia, also known as heartburn or indigestion, is a medical term that describes pain and other symptoms that come from the upper gastro-intestinal (GI) tract (the oesophagus, stomach or duodenum). There are several factors that precipitate dyspepsia, such as eating particular foods, medication, smoking, being overweight and a variety of medical conditions.

The main symptom encountered is usually pain or discomfort in the upper abdomen. Other symptoms that may develop include heartburn (a burning sensation felt in the lower chest area), bloating, belching, quickly feeling full after eating, nausea or vomiting. Care must be taken when treating patients with signs and symptoms related to dyspepsia because the signs and symptoms of a myocardial infarction can be similar.

The symptoms of dyspepsia typically occur in bouts that come and go, rather than being present all the time. Many people have bouts of dyspepsia from time to time. The typical profile encountered is of a person who has dyspeptic symptoms after a large meal. Generally the symptoms subside and do not cause any long-term concern or harm. However, some people have frequent bouts of dyspepsia, which affects their quality of life.

### Medication

There are several medications used to treat dyspepsia. The treatment depends on the causative factors identified and the frequency and intensity of the symptoms the patient encounters.

## Antacids

### Common examples

A range of antacids are available, many as over-the-counter remedies. Products such as Rennie® and Tums® are familiar and can be seen in shops and pharmacies. The most commonly encountered antacid in practice is Gaviscon®.

### Pharmacokinetics and pharmacodynamics

Antacids all act locally (i.e. their site of action is where they are applied). Antacids typically contain a chemical such as aluminium hydroxide, sodium bicarbonate or calcium carbonate, which essentially neutralises stomach acid and allows relief from the symptoms of indigestion. Antacids raise the pH of the stomach (make it less acid) for a relatively short period of time.

Products such as Gaviscon® contain additional ingredients termed **rafting agents**. These sit on top of the contents of the stomach and prevent the acid refluxing (bubbling up) out of the stomach and damaging the oesophagus. This is one source of pain and discomfort felt by patients who suffer from dyspepsia and it can lead to serious long-term problems if left untreated.

### Notable contra-indications/cautions and warnings

Some antacids have significant sodium ($Na^+$) content. This may have a negative influence on those with elevated blood pressure and in medical conditions where sodium intake is restricted.

### Side effects/adverse drug reactions (ADRs)

Aluminium-containing antacids tend to be constipating, and magnesium-containing antacids tend to cause loose stools (laxative effect).

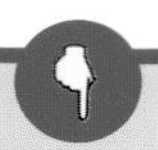

**Clinical pointers**

The fact that antacids neutralise stomach acid means that their administration can affect the absorption of other medication. In many circumstances, antacids should not be administered at the exact same time as other medications.

## Histamine ($H_2$) antagonists

While histamine is more commonly associated with allergic reactions, the $H_2$ histamine receptor subtype is responsible for the control of stomach acid secretion.

### Common examples

The most commonly used $H_2$ antagonist in practice is ranitidine.

### Pharmacokinetics

In treating dyspepsia, these medications can be taken to relieve symptoms when required. However, for the treatment of chronic dyspepsia and stomach ulcers, ranitidine is taken twice daily. If the symptoms of reflux are a problem at night, the daily dose can be taken at night.

### Pharmacodynamics

When histamine receptors are stimulated in the GI tract, they promote the release of acid into the stomach from the parietal cells. This is part of the normal physiology of digestion. $H_2$ antagonists block histamine receptors in the GI tract and this blockade inhibits the release of stomach acid. The lowering of the production of stomach acid provides relief from the symptoms of dyspepsia.

### Side effects/ADRs

The most common side effect of $H_2$-receptor antagonists include diarrhoea, headache and dizziness. Rashes are also noted. As with all medication groups, hypersensitivity to the agent is an important consideration.

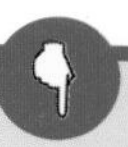

**Clinical pointers**

These medications are available over the counter and from pharmacies. Patients will often self-medicate with $H_2$ antagonists. When asking a patient about the medicines they take, do not forget to ask them about medicines they purchase over the counter.

## Proton pump inhibitors (PPIs)

### Common examples

The most commonly used PPI is omeprazole (Figure 12.1). Others include esomeprazole, rabeprazole, lansoprazole and pantoprazole.

### Pharmacokinetics

Typically, PPIs are taken as a once-daily dose in treating reflux and other conditions. Some PPI formulations will be enterically coated to protect the drug from stomach acid. As such, the capsules should be swallowed whole.

### Pharmacodynamics

PPIs inhibit (block) the proton pump in the parietal cells of the stomach. The proton pump is responsible for 'pumping' $H^+$ ions (acid) into the stomach. The inhibition of the pump raises the pH of the stomach. The decreased acidity provides the relief of symptoms and a chemical environment conducive to the healing of gastric and duodenal ulcers.

### Notable contra-indications/cautions and warnings

Hypersensitivity.

### Side effects/ADRs

Common side effects include GI disturbances and headache.

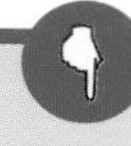

**Clinical pointers**

The presence of any 'alarm symptom' (e.g. significant unintentional weight loss, recurrent vomiting, dysphagia, haematemesis or melena) could be associated with more serious GI conditions.

Many drugs that treat dyspepsia, including $H_2$-receptor antagonists, may mask symptoms of gastric cancer. Continued treatment for dyspepsia requires ongoing appropriate monitoring of the patient.

# 13 Acute diarrhoea and constipation

Figure 13.1 An entry from an in-patient medication chart illustrating the key features to be considered when managing loperamide. Note: this is often a 'when required' medication rather than a regular medication

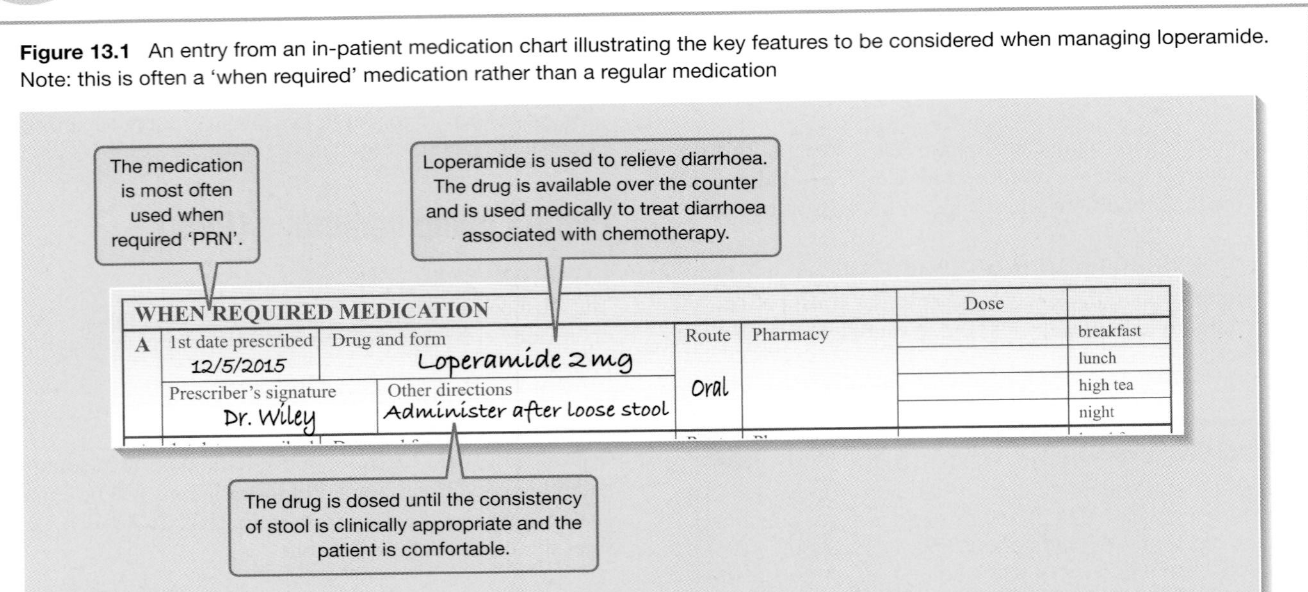

# Acute diarrhoea

## Rehydration

The usual priority in treating acute diarrhoea is the restoration and maintenance of electrolyte balance and hydration. In consequence, most cases of acute diarrhoea are treated using oral rehydration fluids. Severe cases of diarrhoea that cause significant fluid and electrolyte imbalance often require hospitalisation and rapid treatment.

Commonly used rehydration treatments include Dioralyte® and Electrolade®. In addition to the prescribing of these products, they are also available over the counter for self-medication.

## Antimotility agents

In some cases diarrhoea is treated with antimotility drugs (Figure 13.1). These drugs slow down the bowel's peristaltic action, allowing increased water absorption into the body and helping it to produce a more formed stool. The use of antimotility agents is usually confined to acute diarrhoea associated with short-term gastro-intestinal (GI) upset (treatment is **usually** short term and for patient convenience) or to severe diarrhoea caused by chemotherapy. Ongoing diarrhoea associated with chemotherapy can be difficult to manage as well as personally and medically debilitating.

Codeine phosphate, co-phenotrope and loperamide are the most frequently used agents.

## Pharmacokinetics and pharmacodynamics

Codeine phosphate is an opioid agonist and used primarily as an analgesic. Long-term use of opioids like codeine is not recommended because of the potential for misuse. The drug is typically dosed at 30 mg up to four times daily in acute diarrhoea.

Loperamide hydrochloride is also an opioid agonist. The medication acts within 30 minutes to 1 hour of oral administration to slow bowel transit and increase anal sphincter tone (this can be clinically useful in treating faecal incontinence). The speed of onset of action is relevant in using this group of drugs. Although it is an opioid agonist (like morphine and codeine), very little of the drug is absorbed and it does not effectively cross the blood–brain barrier. Therefore, it does not produce the analgesic or euphoric effect of codeine.

Co-phenotrope is a combination of an opioid agonist (diphenoxylate) and an antimuscarinic agent (atropine) that causes a slowing of gut motility.

## Notable contra-indications/cautions and warnings

These drugs are contra-indicated when inhibition of peristalsis of the bowel should be avoided. Co-phenotrope has additional contra-indications and should not be used in conditions where antimuscarinics are contra-indicated (e.g. patients with the condition myasthenia gravis).

These medications are not typically recommended for use in children.

## Side effects

The medications in this group have predictable side effects such as nausea, flatulence and GI discomfort. Co-phenotrope has some antimuscarinic side effects such as dry mouth. Codeine has the same side effects as the other opioid analgesics (see Chapter 23).

# Constipation

## Medication

Most drugs used to treat constipation fall into the following groups. This classification assists with understanding the actions of particular agents but the action of laxatives is complex.

## Bulk-forming laxatives

These drugs act by increasing the bulk of faeces. This stimulates peristalsis in the bowel and facilitates passing stools. Bulk-forming laxatives emulate the role of fibre in the diet. The actions of bulk-forming laxatives may take several days to influence bowel habit. This is an important consideration for both healthcare professionals and patients.

The most commonly used bulk-forming agents include ispaghula husk and methylcellulose. Adequate fluid intake is important with all bulk-forming laxatives; otherwise there is a risk of intestinal obstruction. Side effects include abdominal discomfort and flatulence.

Bulk-forming agents are also used to treat diarrhoea.

## Osmotic laxatives

Osmotic laxatives act by increasing the amount of water present in the large intestine. The most commonly encountered osmotic laxatives are lactulose, macrogols (such as Movicol®) and magnesium hydroxide. Lactulose is a disaccharide that is not absorbed into the circulation from the GI tract. It acts by drawing fluid from the body into the bowel. Lactulose normally takes 48 hours or so to restore bowel action. The drug is also used to treat hepatic encephalopathy.

The macrogols act in a similar manner by increasing stool volume. They are usually administered in a recommended volume of water and this contributes to the action of the agent.

## Stimulant laxatives

Stimulant laxatives directly stimulate intestinal motility. The most frequently encountered examples are senna, bisacodyl, sodium picosulfate and glycerol.

Senna is available as a tablet or a liquid and acts about 8–12 hours after administration. In adult patients, it is administered at night and a bowel movement will occur the following morning. Glycerol is administered as a suppository and has a mildly irritant effect on the GI tract. Stimulant laxatives are often associated with abdominal cramping as one of the more frequent side effects.

## Faecal softeners

Docusate sodium is a faecal softener but also acts as a stimulant laxative. Arachis oil is used as a faecal softener and administered as an enema.

### Clinical pointers

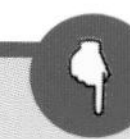

Constipation is a fairly commonly encountered complaint. Accurately diagnosing the cause of constipation is very important to eliminate the possibility that it may be secondary to another illness or disease process.

Bowel habit can vary significantly from person to person. Many patients have beliefs about 'normal' bowel habit that result in the improper use of laxatives. Laxatives can also be misused as a means to control weight in conditions such as anorexia nervosa.

Arachis oil is a peanut oil and while it is **unlikely** to trigger an allergic response in sensitive patients, the potential risk should always be considered.

# 14 Chronic bowel disease

Figure 14.1 An entry from an in-patient medication chart illustrating how Asacol MR may be prescribed and some key features to be considered when it is administered

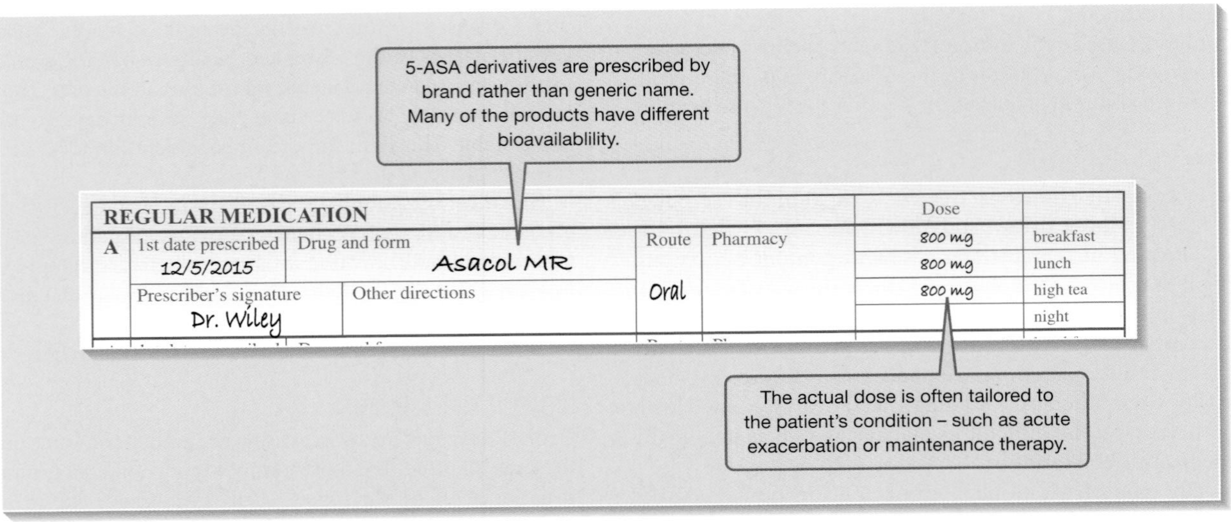

This chapter focuses on the medicines management of inflammatory bowel disease (IBD). The medications discussed will typically be used to treat Crohn's disease and ulcerative colitis (Figure 14.1).

## Medications

Aminosalicylates, corticosteroids and immunoregulating agents are the most frequently used drugs to treat IBD. Many medications used in IBD can be administered locally and/or systemically; this is usually dependent on the patient's diagnosis, response to treatment and which part of the gastro-intestinal (GI) tract is affected.

## Aminosalicylates

These medicines are essentially anti-inflammatory compounds with similar structures to aspirin. There are four commonly used aminosalicylates that contain the compound 5-aminosalicylic acid (5-ASA): sulfasalazine, mesalazine, balsalzide and olsalazine.

### Posology, pharmacokinetics and pharmacodynamics

This group of medicines are available as oral medications, enemas, foam enemas (which are useful for patients who have problems retaining other types of enema), powders and suppositories. Doses found in the drug literature often refer to acute treatment dosage regimes (for use when the disease flares up and symptoms are at their worst) and maintenance therapy regimes (when the disease is less active).

### Notable contra-indications/cautions and warnings

Patients taking the 5-ASA derivatives require blood tests to monitor renal function at regular intervals during treatment. The 5-ASA compounds should not be used when a patient has a hypersensitivity to salicylate compounds.

### Side effects and adverse drug reactions (ADRs)

The most common side effects encountered include GI upset, headache and rash. Patients should be carefully observed and counselled regarding any unexplained bleeding, bruising, sore throats and malaise that occur during treatment because this may be indicative of a blood disorder related to 5-ASA therapy. A full blood count needs to be performed if these symptoms arise, and if there is evidence of a blood dyscrasia (an abnormal 'balance' of the cells present in blood) the drug should be discontinued.

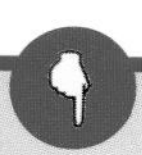

**Clinical pointers**

Many 5-ASA-based oral medications are specially coated to release their active ingredients in a particular part of the GI tract. These are termed 'modified-release (MR) tablets'. It is important that these tablets are swallowed whole and not broken or chewed at the point of administration.

There are many branded products containing the medication mesalazine. The drug delivery characteristics of oral mesalazine preparations may vary. While it is generally evidenced that no one preparation is better than another, **if the preparation is changed, patients may report changes in efficacy of the therapy**.

## Corticosteroids

Corticosteroids are used in many clinical contexts including the treatment of IBD. They are sometimes used alone but more often in combination with 5-ASA compounds. They are used as short-course adjunct therapies and also as longer-term treatments.

### Posology, pharmacokinetics and pharmacodynamics

Corticosteroids are most frequently administered by the oral route (e.g. prednisolone and budesonide) and the rectal route (e.g. hydrocortisone and budesonide). In more severe cases and exacerbations of disease, corticosteroids such as hydrocortisone and methylprednisolone are administered intravenously.

Corticosteroids are anti-inflammatory compounds. They are believed to regulate a variety of cellular functions leading to suppression of immunological function and, as a result, an improvement in the symptoms of IBD.

### Notable contra-indications/cautions and warnings

There are guidelines available to ensure that steroids are stopped appropriately, because the withdrawal of steroids can lead to adverse events.

### Side effects/ADRs

The side effects associated with steroid use are numerous because of the variety of actions steroids have on physiological function. A comprehensive list of side effects can be found in the British National Formulary (BNF), the summary of product characteristics or the patient information leaflet for the prescribed medication.

Prolonged treatment with corticosteroids can cause the adrenal gland to atrophy and can affect its ability to produce endogenous steroids. Other adverse effects include increased susceptibility to infection, euphoria, nightmares and labile mood.

## Immunoregulating agents

There are numerous drugs used to treat IBD that modulate the body's immune response. These drugs, like the steroids, may be used in several medical conditions, not only IBD. It is important that as a nurse you understand the nature of the patient's illness and how the drug is being used. Azathioprine, ciclosporin, mercaptopurine and methotrexate have been identified and have evidenced roles in treating IBD.

In addition to the medications discussed earlier, the monoclonal antibody therapies infliximab, adalimumab and golimumab are used to treat IBD. They are often used in specific phases of the diseases (e.g. acute exacerbations) and most often when patients are unable to tolerate other therapies or their disease does not respond to other therapies.

### Posology and use in practice

The principal action of these drugs is to dampen the immune response that is believed to be one key causative factor in IBD. These drugs are usually used in severe ulcerative colitis and 'unresponsive'/chronically active Crohn's disease.

These medications are immunosuppressive in nature and this can lead to short-term and potential long-term adverse events. The monoclonal antibody therapies are relatively recent additions to the list of drugs used to treat IBD. Owing to their relatively expensive drug and monitoring costs, these drugs are subject to technology appraisals undertaken by the National Institute for Health and Care Excellence (NICE).

### Activity

Many immunosuppressants, such as ciclosporin, are prescribed by brand to ensure that the plasma concentration of these important drugs remains as steady as possible.

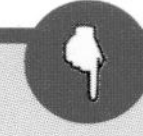

**Clinical pointers**

More potent agents like the immunosuppressants are dosed by body weight rather than by a 'flat' dose or age-based dose. Check calculations carefully!

# Nausea and vomiting

Figure 15.1 An entry from an in-patient medication chart illustrating how metoclopramide may be prescribed and some key features to be considered when it is administered

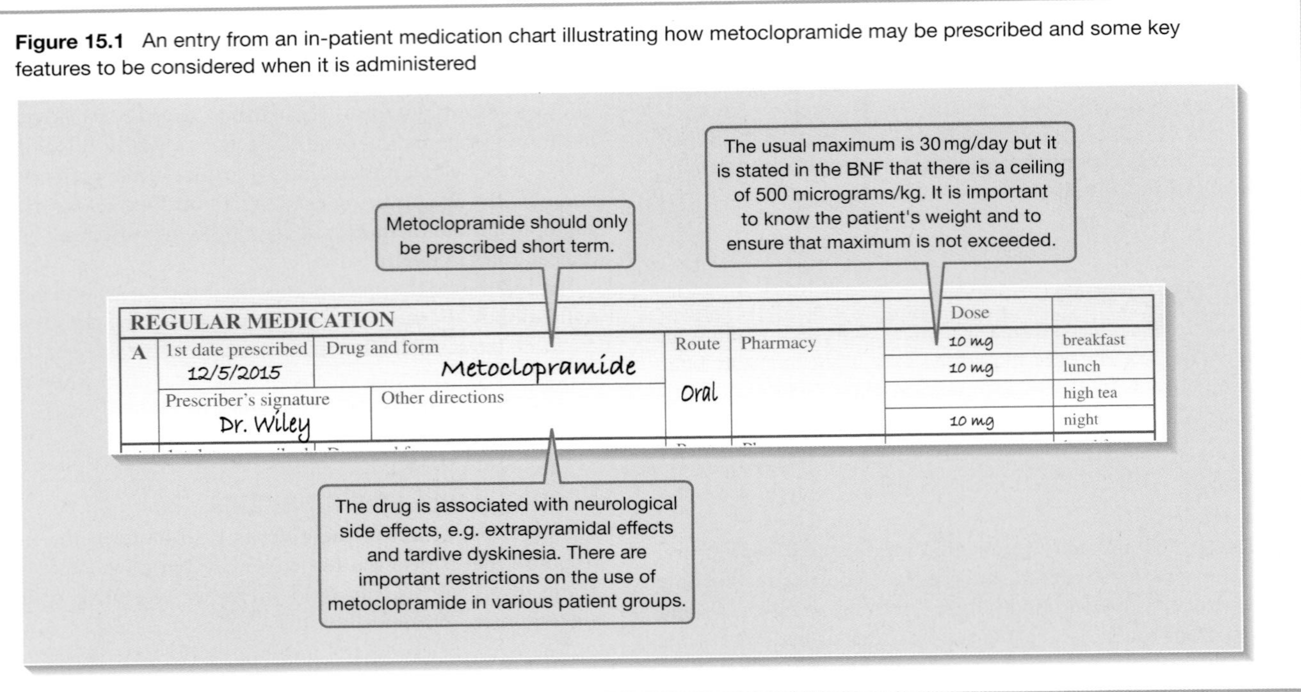


There are many circumstances when medication in practice may be used to manage nausea and vomiting (Figure 15.1). There are a wide range of causes of nausea and vomiting (e.g. migraine, gastro-intestinal [GI] infection, pregnancy, emetogenic chemotherapy, tumours, motion sickness, medication overdose and side effects). While the nausea and vomiting themselves can be treated, in most cases it is important to identify the cause and treat the underlying problem.

## Medications

The most commonly prescribed anti-emetics include metoclopramide and domperidone, antihistamines (e.g. cyclizine) and 5-$HT_3$ receptor antagonists (e.g. ondansetron).

## Metoclopramide

Metoclopramide and domperidone have similar mechanisms of action, but their use in practice is subtly different. The drugs are used for nausea and vomiting associated with chemotherapy, radiotherapy, post-operatively and in assisting with conditions in which gastric emptying is slower (e.g. migraine).

### Posology, pharmacokinetics and pharmacodynamics

Metoclopramide is given by mouth (tablet or oral solution) or via the injectable route. There are specific guidelines for the use of metoclopramide in the British National Formulary (BNF), the summary of product characteristics (SPC) and any literature that refers to metoclopramide dosing.

The drug is usually dosed three times daily and is also used as a once-only dose for procedures such as barium swallow and meal. It reaches its peak plasma concentration about 1 hour after oral dosing. The drug's elimination is slowed by renal impairment and it is excreted into breast milk.

Metoclopramide acts by encouraging peristalsis (especially in the upper GI tract) and speeding up gastric emptying (prokinetic activity). Its action is related to its blockade of dopamine receptors that influence gastric motility and the trigger threshold of the chemo-receptor trigger zone (CTZ).

### Notable contra-indications/cautions and warnings

Cautions include use in elderly people, young adults and children, atopic allergy and certain cardiac conduction disturbances

*Medicines Management for Nurses at a Glance*. First Edition. Simon Young and Ben Pitcher. © 2016 John Wiley & Sons, Ltd. Published 2016 by John Wiley & Sons, Ltd.
www.ataglanceseries.com/nursing/medicinesmanagement

as the drug can interact with other medicines that interfere with cardiac rhythm.

The drug is contra-indicated in GI obstruction, GI perforation or GI haemorrhage. Use of the drug post-GI surgery and in the condition phaeochromocytoma is also a contra-indication.

The blockade of dopamine receptors by metoclopramide can exacerbate or mask the symptoms of conditions that are caused by deterioration of the dopaminergic pathways (e.g. Parkinson's disease).

### Side effects/adverse drug reactions (ADRs)

There is a Medicines and Healthcare Products Regulatory Agency (MHRA)/Commission on Human Medicines (CHM) advice warning in the BNF on the restriction of the use of metoclopramide. This relates to a risk of neurological side effects in certain groups of patients, and imposes restrictions on doses and duration of use.

The most worrying side effect includes extrapyramidal symptoms (parkinsonism). Other side effects including drowsiness, diarrhoea, restlessness and anxiety are reported. The drug can cause QT prolongation (after intravenous administration) and galactorrhoea, and it is one of the drugs known to cause gynaecomastia.

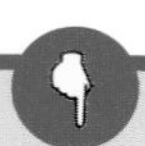

**Clinical pointers**

Metoclopramide is included in compound preparations, with medications like paracetamol, as a way of administering an analgesic and an anti-emetic in one dose for conditions such as migraine. Domperidone does not cross the blood–brain barrier so does not have the same central effects associated with using metoclopramide. Its actions are similar but each clinical situation dictates the choice and suitability of the drug.

## Antihistamines

One of the most commonly prescribed antihistamines used for nausea and vomiting is cyclizine. Cinnarizine and promethazine are used to treat vestibular disorder and to prevent and treat motion sickness.

### Posology, pharmacokinetics and pharmacodynamics

Cyclizine is administered orally, intravenously, intramuscularly or by subcutaneous injection (via a syringe driver). In palliative care settings, it is delivered continuously alongside opiate analgesics and other agents to counteract the nausea induced by the opiates. It is not fully understood how antihistamines act to treat nausea and vomiting.

### Notable contra-indications/cautions and warnings

Cyclizine is a medication that has been misused for its euphoric and psychoactive effects. It has antimuscarinic effects, which means that it should be used cautiously with patients who have glaucoma or prostatic hypertrophy. It can cause a fall in cardiac output and hence should also be used cautiously in those with severe heart failure.

The drug causes variable degrees of drowsiness that should be considered when caring for patients.

### Side effects/ADRs

ADRs include headache, psychomotor impairment and antimuscarinic effects (see earlier) – for example, dry mouth, blurred vision and GI disturbances.

## 5-HT$_3$ receptor antagonists

The 5-HT$_3$ receptor antagonists are used primarily in controlling nausea and vomiting post-operatively or associated with chemotherapy.

### Posology, pharmacokinetics and pharmacodynamics

Ondansetron is available as tablets and in liquid, orodispersible and injectable dosage forms. The options are important when vomiting is present and the swallowing of solid oral dosage forms may not be possible. In some situations, such as after an operation or the administration of cytotoxic chemotherapeutic drugs, the GI tract releases 5-HT (also called serotonin) that initiates a reflex that can trigger nausea and vomiting. Ondansetron and its analogues block the 5-HT and thereby prevent this reflex.

### Notable contra-indications/cautions and warnings

Congenital long QT syndrome and any factors that cause QT interval prolongation.

### Side effects/ADRs

Please see the BNF and SPC for specific lists.

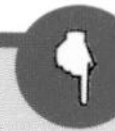

**Clinical pointers**

Other medications are also used to treat nausea and vomiting: drugs like nabilone, aprepitant and members of the phenothiazine family (e.g. prochlorperazine). Each drug has its own clinical circumstance in which it is the most suitable. Prochlorperazine, for example, is available in a buccal form that bypasses the need to swallow medication. Cannabaniod derivatives (nabilone) and the neurokinin receptor antagonists (aprepitant and fosaprepitant) are typically used when other drugs have failed to control vomiting caused by chemotherapy.

# Anti-anginals

Figure 16.1 An entry from an in-patient medication chart illustrating how anti-anginals may be prescribed and some key features to be considered when it is administered

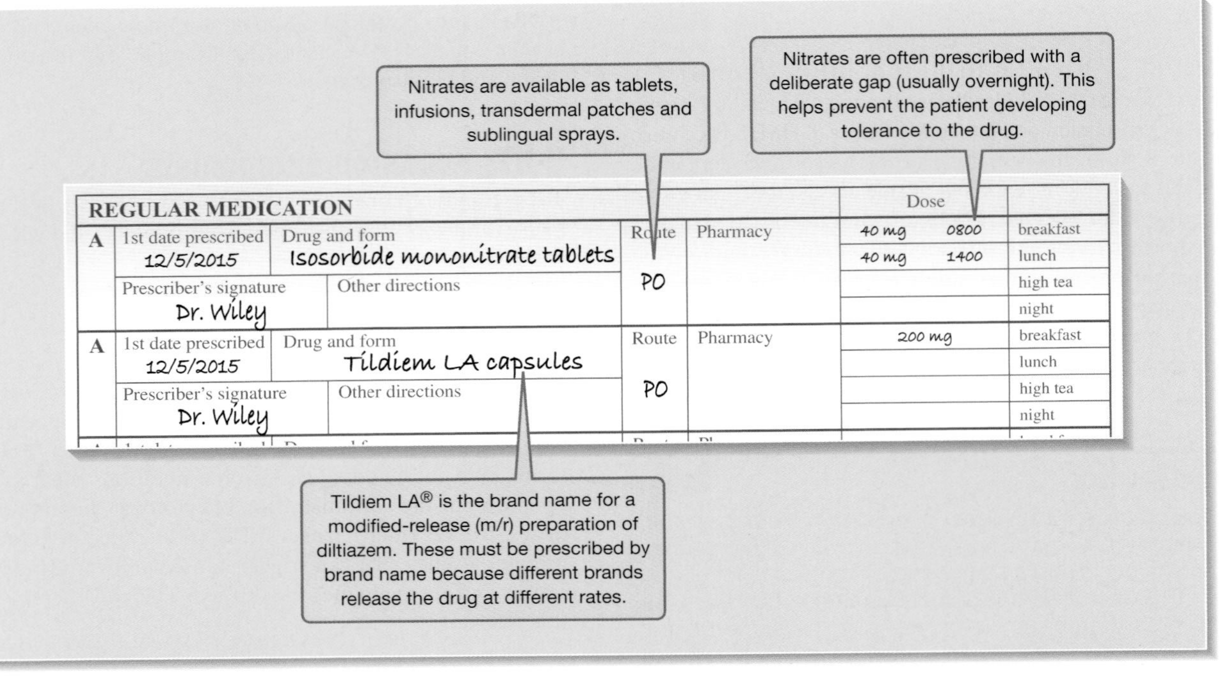


These are drugs used to prevent and relieve angina (Figure 16.1).

## Indications

Angina pectoris (angina) is a crushing vice-like pain, felt across a person's chest and left shoulder, caused by a lack of oxygen to the heart. It is mainly caused by coronary heart disease, which results in narrowing of the blood vessels. Unlike skeletal muscle, which, when starved of oxygen, can 'go to sleep' and survive for many hours, cardiac cells cannot switch off and will remain active despite an insufficient supply of oxygen. This anaerobic respiration will quickly damage and eventually kill the myocytes, resulting in a heart attack (myocardial infarction).

Angina is the result of insufficient blood (and the oxygen it carries) reaching the heart to meet the demand placed upon it. The harder the heart works, the more oxygen it requires (this is why angina is often triggered by exertion).

The drugs used to treat angina work in two main ways:

- Increasing the blood (and oxygen) supply to the heart.
- Reducing the oxygen demand of the heart.

## Nitrates

Nitrates are the most commonly encountered treatment for angina. They trigger the vasodilation of blood vessels, allowing easier passage of blood to the heart and lowering the blood pressure. This lowering in blood pressure reduces the workload of the heart. These drugs are therefore successful in increasing the supply of oxygenated blood to the heart **and** reducing the oxygen demand of the heart.

### Common examples

- Glyceryl trinitrate.
- Isosorbide mononitrate.
- Isosorbide dinitrate.

### Pharmacodynamics

In the normal functioning of blood vessels, the innermost layer of the vessel wall (the tunica intima) is made up of endothelial cells. These are able to produce a signalling molecule called nitric oxide (NO), which causes a relaxation in the smooth muscle of the vascular wall. This helps the vessel to dilate (widen or expand)

and allow more blood to flow through it. When nitrates enter the body they are broken down into NO, hijacking this control mechanism and causing widespread vasodilation.

### Pharmacokinetics

Nitrates can come in a variety of forms, and are used in different situations. These are essentially different ways of delivering nitrates to the body, although in the end they lead to the formation of an excess of NO.

### Glyceryl tri-nitrate (GTN)

GTN is a nitrate that comes in a liquid form that is usually sprayed under the tongue. This form of nitrate is the most easily recognised and is the form used by patients to relieve an angina attack. The sublingual route is very fast acting and therefore ideal for the rapid relief of symptoms.

### Isosorbide mononitrates

Isosorbide mononitrate (ISMN) is a nitrate that is delivered orally in tablet form. The tablets release the nitrates into the blood stream gradually throughout the day. They are used to protect against angina attacks rather than to treat an attack in progress.

The body quickly adapts to continuous stimuli; if blood vessels are continuously exposed to nitrates, they quickly desensitise and you see a reduced response to the medication. To try and prevent this, the dosing regimen for nitrate tablets may be altered. Typically, we try and administer drugs regularly through the day with no large gaps; this helps keep the concentrations of drugs in the blood as stable as possible. With nitrates, the regimen is sometimes set up to give a longer gap through the night, allowing the nitrate concentration to fall when the patient is asleep and therefore least likely to have an angina attack. This gap helps prevent tolerance to the nitrates.

### Isosorbide dinitrate

This nitrate is available in a variety of forms, but is most commonly used as a solution (Isoket®) administered intravenously (in hospital) in very severe cases.

### Notable contraindications/cautions and warnings

There are a range of cautions associated with nitrates (see the British National Formulary [BNF]). Many are associated with the sudden and substantial drop in blood pressure that can result from taking the drug.

### Side effects/adverse drug reactions (ADRs)

The sudden drop in blood pressure can cause postural hypotension and dizziness. Other side effects include flushing, syncope and headache.

## Calcium channel blockers

- Diltiazem.
- Verapamil.
- Dihydropyridines:
  - Nifedipine
  - Nimodipine
  - Amlodipine.

### Pharmacodynamics

Calcium ions play an important role in the activation of muscle contraction in the heart and vasculature, and in the conduction of electrical signals from cell to cell within the heart. The calcium ions enter the cells through ion channels (Chapter 10). Calcium channel blockers block these ion channels, thereby reducing muscle contraction in the vasculature, which causes dilation, and slowing the conduction through the heart. The vasodilation reduces blood pressure and eases the flow of blood to the heart. The effect on cardiac conduction slows the heart, reducing its demand for oxygen.

Some calcium channel blockers act primarily on the heart (diltiazem and verapamil), while others have a greater effect on the vasculature (dihydropyridines).

### Pharmacokinetics

Calcium channel blockers are predominantly administered in oral dosage forms, including some formulations that are modified release. However, some can be given intravenously.

### Notable contra-indications/cautions and warnings

Diltiazem and verapamil reduce the speed of conduction through the heart and so it is possible that they can cause distinct drops in cardiac output, precipitating heart failure.

### Side effects/ADRs

Calcium channels are found throughout the body on a variety on different tissues. Therefore, blocking them can have a wide range of side effects: most commonly, nausea and abdominal discomfort; heart palpitations, flushing, oedema; headache, dizziness, sleep disturbances and fatigue.

# Anti-arrhythmics

**Figure 17.1** An entry from an in-patient medication chart illustrating how some common anti-arrhythmic drugs may be prescribed and some key features to be considered when they are administered

Amiodarone has a number of side effects that include phototoxic reactions causing a discolouration of the skin.

| REGULAR MEDICATION | | | | | Dose | |
|---|---|---|---|---|---|---|
| A | 1st date prescribed<br>12/5/2015 | Drug and form<br>Amiodarone tablets | Route | Pharmacy | 200 mg | breakfast |
| | | | | | 200 mg | lunch |
| | Prescriber's signature<br>Dr. Wiley | Other directions<br>Avoid direct sunlight<br>Wear sunscreen | Oral | | 200 mg | high tea |
| | | | | | | night |

| REGULAR MEDICATION | | | | | Dose | |
|---|---|---|---|---|---|---|
| A | 1st date prescribed<br>12/5/2015 | Drug and form<br>Digoxin tablet | Route | Pharmacy | 62.5 micrograms | breakfast |
| | | | | | | lunch |
| | Prescriber's signature<br>Dr. Wiley | Other directions<br>Do not administer if HR<60 | Oral | | | high tea |
| | | | | | | night |

Digoxin will lower the heart rate. If the heart rate drops below 60 it can be harmful to continue with treatment.

Micrograms should always be written in full and not abbreviated to 'mcg' or 'µg'.

A healthy heart should beat in a regular pattern and at a reasonable speed, beating faster at times of high demand and slower at times of rest. If the heart beats in an abnormal fashion, it is said to have an arrhythmia. This can relate to the heart beating at an irregular rate, irregular strength, very fast (tachycardia) or very slow (bradycardia). While some patients may live with an arrhythmia without any serious symptoms, others may experience palpitations, dizziness or even blackouts. Some arrhythmias can be life threatening, disrupting the normal functioning of the heart to such a degree that cardiac output is insufficient to support life. Additionally, in some arrhythmias such as atrial fibrillation (AF), blood is not cleared adequately from the chambers of the heart, resulting in the formation of clots that can precipitate pulmonary embolisms and strokes.

There are a number of drugs that are used to treat arrhythmias (Figure 17.1).

## Digoxin

Digoxin (a cardiac glycoside) is one of the most common anti-arrhythmic agents used. It is effective but has an array of side effects.

### Indications

Useful in treating a variety of arrhythmias, including AF and atrial flutter, and has the effect of slowing and strengthening the beat of the heart.

### Pharmacodynamics

The normal electrical activity of the heart is controlled by sodium ($Na^+$) and potassium ($K^+$). These ions are moved into and out of the cardiac myocyte using a transport protein called $K^+/Na^+$ ATPase that sits in the cell membrane. Digoxin acts on this protein, affecting the balance of ions within the cell and the electrical activity.

### Pharmacokinetics

Digoxin can be given intravenously but is more commonly taken in tablet form. It can be used in the treatment of an acute episode of arrhythmia or as a long-term treatment. It is excreted by the kidneys, and can therefore build up to toxic levels if renal function is impaired.

### Notable contra-indications/cautions and warnings

Digoxin's mechanism of action involves interacting with the protein $K^+/Na^+$ ATPase. Having too much potassium (hyperkalaemia) or too little potassium (hypokalaemia) in the body will affect the action of digoxin and increase the likelihood of toxicity.

Common causes of hypokalaemia include diarrhoea and vomiting and the use of some diuretics (e.g. furosemide), while other cardiac drugs (such as Angiotensin converting enzyme inhibitors) may cause hyperkalaemia.

### Side effects/adverse drug reactions (ADRs)

Digoxin has a number of side effects that can cause a patient difficulties.

Although intended to treat arrhythmias, it can also cause arrhythmias! Other symptoms include nausea, diarrhoea, xanthopsia (yellowing of the eyesight) and gynaecomastia (the development of breasts in men). Patients can also develop confusion and agitation.

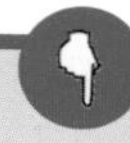

**Clinical pointers**

It is tricky to get the dosing right for digoxin because it has a narrow therapeutic window (i.e. there is only a small difference between an effective dose and a toxic dose). To try and avoid accidental overdosing, patients have blood tests often to check their digoxin levels.

Digoxin overdose can be very serious. A drug has been developed that helps clear digoxin from the body. This is called a digoxin-specific antibody (DigiFab®).

## Amiodarone

### Indications

This can be used for acute and prophylactic treatment of atrial and ventricular arrhythmias.

### Pharmacodynamics

Amiodarone affects the movement of sodium and potassium into the cardiac myocytes. It also acts on the sympathetic nervous system (SNS) reducing the effects of adrenaline and noradrenaline. This slows down the speed of conduction of the electrical impulses and reduces the frequency in which cells can be activated. This helps slow and strengthen the rhythm of the heart.

### Pharmacokinetics

Amiodarone can be administered orally or by intravenous injection (which acts rapidly). It has a long half-life (i.e. it remains in the body for a long time). Patients are often started on a higher dose of amiodarone as a loading dose to get the plasma concentrations up to the required level. Then a lower 'maintenance' dose is given to maintain the plasma concentration at that level for longer periods of treatment.

### Side effects/ADRs

Although effective at resolving arrhythmias, amiodarone comes with several notable side effects. These include photosensitive rashes (patients must stay out of the sun) and grey/blue discolouration of the skin that can be quite disfiguring. Many patients develop corneal deposits that can cause dazzling of the eyesight at night. Patients can also develop problems with thyroid function, or respiratory, hepatic and neurological symptoms.

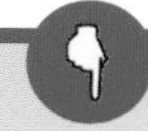

**Clinical pointers**

Because of the potential damaging effects of amiodarone, a patient should have their liver and thyroid function checked before commencing treatment and every 6 months thereafter.

## Other anti-arrhythmic drugs

### Beta-blockers

Although primarily associated with reducing blood pressure (see Chapter 19), beta-blockers can also reduce the excitability of the heart muscle, arrhythmias and ectopic beats. Adrenaline lowers the threshold of stimulation for a cardiac cell to fire off an action potential, making an ectopic beat or arrhythmia more likely. It is in part through this mechanism that arrhythmias can be exacerbated through stress. Blocking the receptor with a beta-blocker prevents this effect.

There is a range of other anti-arrhythmics available. Examples include flecainide, lignocaine, adenosine and mexiletine. These can be used in a variety of clinical situations to deal with very specific types of arrhythmia.

# 18 Heart failure

Figure 18.1 An entry from an in-patient medication chart illustrating how some drugs used in heart failure may be prescribed and some key features to be considered when they are administered

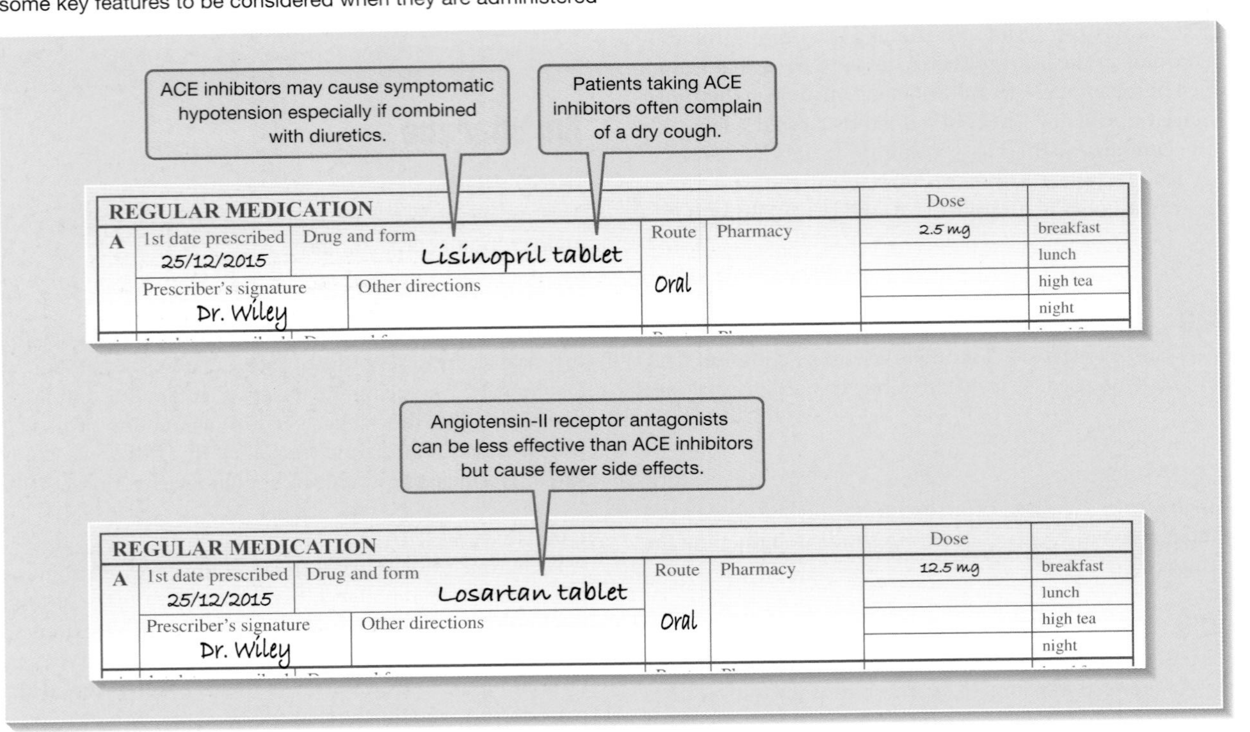

Heart failure occurs when the heart becomes damaged and loses its ability to adequately supply the organs and tissues of the body with blood. When we describe heart failure, it does not mean that the heart has totally failed but that it is failing to provide the necessary output.

The body will use the renin-angiotensin system to increase blood pressure to improve the supply of blood to the tissues. It does this through a number of processes including increasing thirst to retain more fluid, thus increasing circulating volume, causing peripheral vasoconstriction, and thickening the muscle layer of the heart and vasculature. If you had low blood pressure due to dehydration or blood loss, these processes would be important steps in restoring blood volume and blood pressure. However, these processes put extra strain on the heart. If the heart is damaged, this extra strain can increase the degree of failure, which in turn triggers more adaptation. This cycle continues: the body struggling to maintain blood pressure and trying to compensate by retaining more and more fluid, thereby raising blood pressure, bringing about oedema, fatigue and breathlessness. If untreated, this cycle can lead to death.

To treat heart failure, we use drugs that interfere with these adaptive processes and therefore prevent the retention of fluid and rising of blood pressure (Figure 18.1). While we are discussing these drugs in the context of the treatment of heart failure, they can also be used in the treatment of hypertension.

## Angiotensin converting enzyme (ACE) inhibitors

ACE inhibitors can often be identified by the name ending they share – **pril**.

### Common examples

- Lisinopril.
- Ramipril.
- Enalapril.
- Perindopril.

### Indications

ACE inhibitors can be used in all forms of heart failure, often in conjunction with other drugs. They are also used in the treatment of hypertension.

### Pharmacodynamics

As discussed in Chapters 10 and 11, many processes within the body are controlled by signalling molecules such as hormones or neurotransmitters that trigger tissues or organs to create effects. In the processes involved in heart failure, one of the key hormones is angiotensin-II. When blood pressure drops, sympathetic stimulation triggers the kidney to secrete a hormone called renin; this acts on a protein called angiotensinogen, converting it into the inactive angiotensin-I. This in turn is converted by ACE into the active angiotensin-II.

Angiotensin-II formation triggers vasoconstriction, thickening of the muscle layer of the heart and fluid retention. This will cause a further decline in heart function and worsening of symptoms. Inhibiting the action of the ACE prevents the conversion of angiotensin-I into angiotensin-II and thereby all the subsequent processes.

### Pharmacokinetics

ACE inhibitors are administered orally and absorbed into the blood at a moderate pace, reaching peak concentrations in the blood 7 hours after administration. However, despite the relatively quick rate of absorption, patients may not experience any symptomatic benefit immediately.

### Notable contra-indications/cautions and warnings

Because ACE inhibitors prevent water retention (essentially increasing fluid output), they should be used with caution in those who are dehydrated or hypovolaemic.

### Side effects/adverse drug reactions (ADRs)

ACE inhibitors may result in a significant lowering of blood pressure that can result in dizziness or even fainting.

ACE inhibitors are not completely 'specific': they can inhibit the action of other enzymes as well. In particular, they have been found to inhibit the enzyme kininase II. This enzyme normally breaks down bradykinin (an inflammatory mediator); the resulting build-up of bradykinin can cause sensations of itching and irritation, and most notably manifests as an irritating, dry cough.

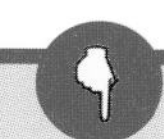

**Clinical pointers**

Because ACE inhibitors can cause notable drops in blood pressure, it can be important to keep a close eye on patients who have just started them and to advise them of the possibility that they may become dizzy when they stand up. They may even require some help and support when mobilising. ACE inhibitors can also have an effect on renal function that can result in hyperkalaemia. This usually requires monitoring and needs to be considered if the patient is taking any other medication that can cause hyperkalaemia, such as potassium-sparing diuretics (Chapter 20). Additionally, the action of other cardiac drugs such as digoxin can be disrupted by deranged electrolytes.

## Angiotensin-II receptor antagonists

These are also known as angiotensin receptor blockers (ARBs).

ARBs can often be identified by the name ending they share – **artan**.

### Common examples

- Irbesartan.
- Valsartan.
- Losartan.

### Pharmacodynamics

As discussed earlier, the actions of angiotensin-II are key factors in the disease process of heart failure. Angiotensin-II binds to a receptor that is present in many organs and tissues. ARBs antagonise (block) this receptor. This prevents the angiotensin-II from binding and therefore prevents the vasoconstriction and fluid retention.

### Side effects/ADRs

Similar to ACE inhibitors, angiotensin-II receptor antagonists can cause hypotension and hyperkalaemia. However, because they do not inhibit the ACE, they also do not inhibit the kininase II and therefore do not cause the dry cough.

## Other drugs used in heart failure

Heart failure is a complex problem that involves a number of physiological control mechanisms. As such, there are a number of different therapeutic drugs that can be used to try and control the disease process. These include diuretics to reduce fluid retention and lower blood pressure, and other antihypertensives (which will be discussed in depth in their own chapters).

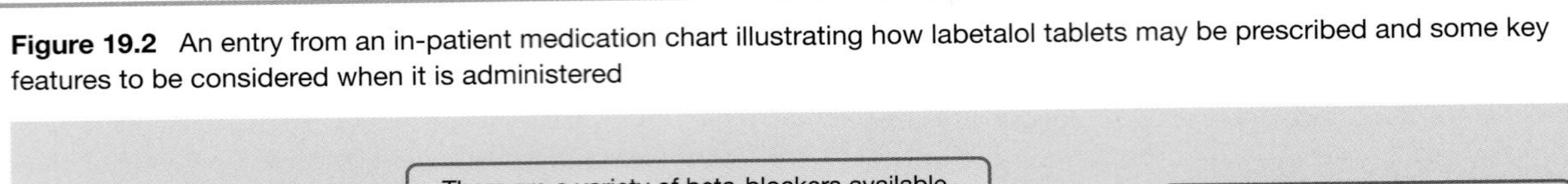

# 19 Hypertension

Figure 19.2 An entry from an in-patient medication chart illustrating how labetalol tablets may be prescribed and some key features to be considered when it is administered

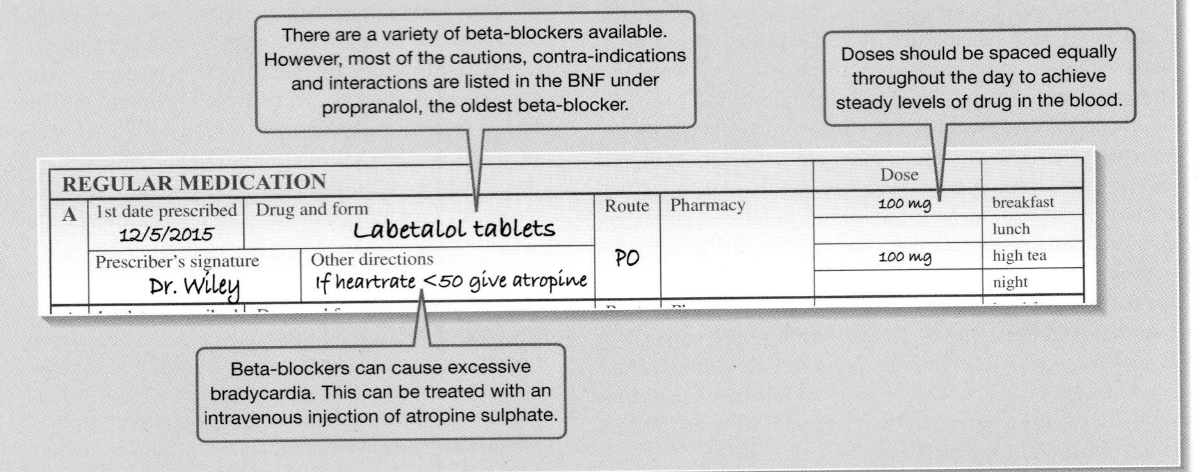

# Drugs used to treat hypertension

It is a well-known fact that having high blood pressure (hypertension) is bad for your health and increases your risk of numerous health complaints. Blood pressure is controlled by a number of different physiological mechanisms that raise or lower the blood pressure in response to physiological requirement or to pathological disease processes (Figure 19.1). Interfering with these mechanisms allows us to override the body's control and return the blood pressure to safer levels.

Blood pressure is the force the blood exerts on the walls of blood vessels; it is caused by the outflow of blood from the heart meeting resistance as it tries to flow through the ever smaller branches of the vasculature.

As such, blood pressure can be described by the equation:

Blood pressure (BP) = cardiac output (CO) × peripheral resistance (PR)

To alter a patient's blood pressure, a drug must affect either the CO or the PR.

## Beta-blockers

These can often be identified by the name ending they share – **lol** (Figure 19.1).

### Common examples

- Atenolol.
- Propranolol.
- Labetalol.
- Carvedilol.

### Pharmacodynamics

One of the most important mechanisms the body uses for the control of blood pressure is the sympathetic nervous system (SNS). Among its many functions, the SNS raises the blood pressure by stimulating the heart, vasculature and kidneys with adrenaline (epinephrine) and noradrenaline (norepinephrine). These agents bind to specific receptors (Chapter 10) on the cell membranes of the target tissue. When bound to, these receptors trigger a physiological action, which acts to raise the blood pressure by increasing CO and/or PR (increased heart rate, vasoconstriction, increased fluid retention). The receptors on the different tissues are subtly different. For example, the subtype of receptor found on the heart is the $beta_1$ adrenergic receptor. These differences in receptor subtype can be pharmacologically exploited.

The beta-blockers act by blocking beta adrenergic receptors with the intention of preventing the sympathetic stimulation of the heart (and thereby any rise in blood pressure) but not interfering with the role of the SNS elsewhere in the body.

### Notable contraindications/cautions and warnings

As discussed earlier, beta-blockers prevent the binding of adrenaline and noradrenaline to the $beta_1$ adrenergic receptors on the heart. While their action is intended to be specific to these $beta_1$ receptors, they can also block $beta_2$ receptors found on the lungs. When stimulated, $beta_2$ receptors cause bronchodilation (a relaxation of the smooth muscle lining the small airways, which facilitates easier movement of air into the lungs). This mechanism is used in the treatment of asthma where drugs like salbutamol are $beta_2$ agonists that trigger bronchodilation. Because beta-blockers can block $beta_2$ receptors, they can precipitate bronchospasm and block the action of drugs like salbutamol. As such, beta-blockers should usually be avoided in patients with a history of asthma.

### Side effects/adverse drug reactions (ADRs)

Beta-blockers may result in a significant lowering of blood pressure that could result in dizziness or even fainting. This can even occur if the blood pressure of the patient is above 'normal' but lower than what the patient's body has been used to.

Bradycardia (low heart rate) – blocking adrenaline and noradrenaline from having an effect on the heart will also slow the heart rate.

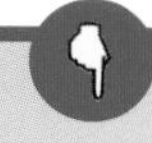

**Clinical pointers**

***Recommendation for patients***

*Warning: do not stop taking this medicine unless your doctor tells you to stop.*

The body will always try and adapt to changes forced upon it. In response to adrenergic receptors being blocked by beta-blockers, the body will increase the number of receptors on that tissue. If a patient suddenly stops taking the beta-blockers, then the body's adrenaline will be able to bind the increased number of receptors causing an increased response.

The upshot of this is that suddenly stopping beta-blockers will cause the blood pressure to rise and put the patient in a more unsafe position than before they started treatment. Therefore, beta-blockers should always be reduced in stages before discontinuation.

## Calcium channel blockers

Calcium channel blockers prevent the entry of calcium into cardiac and smooth muscle cells. This has the effect of reducing the contractility of the muscle and the speed of conduction of action potentials across them. Some calcium channel blockers act more predominantly on the heart muscle, reducing CO. Others act more predominantly on the peripheral vasculature, reducing vasoconstriction and therefore PR (for more on calcium channel blockers, see Chapter 16).

## Angiotensin converting enzyme (ACE) inhibitors and angiotensin receptor blockers (ARBS)

While often seen as a treatment for heart failure, these are also used in treating hypertension. By disrupting the renin-angiotensin system, they prevent vasoconstriction and reduce secretion of aldosterone and antidiuretic hormone. This reduces fluid retention, decreasing CO and PR (for more on ACE inhibitors and ARBs, see Chapter 18).

## Diuretics

Diuretics increase fluid output, thus reducing circulating volume. Reducing the amount of fluid within a system will reduce its pressure (much like letting air out of a balloon). Reducing the circulating volume also reduces the venous return (the flow of blood back to the heart) because the heart cannot pump out more blood than is returned to it; reducing venous return reduces CO and therefore blood pressure (for more on diuretics, see Chapter 20).

## Other drugs used in hypertension

There are a variety of drugs used in the treatment of high blood pressure that act on different aspects of the cardiovascular system to reduce either CO or PR. Information about these less commonly used drugs can be found in the British National Formulary (BNF).

# 20 Diuretics

Figure 20.1 An entry from an in-patient medication chart illustrating how diuretics may be prescribed and some key features to be considered when it is administered

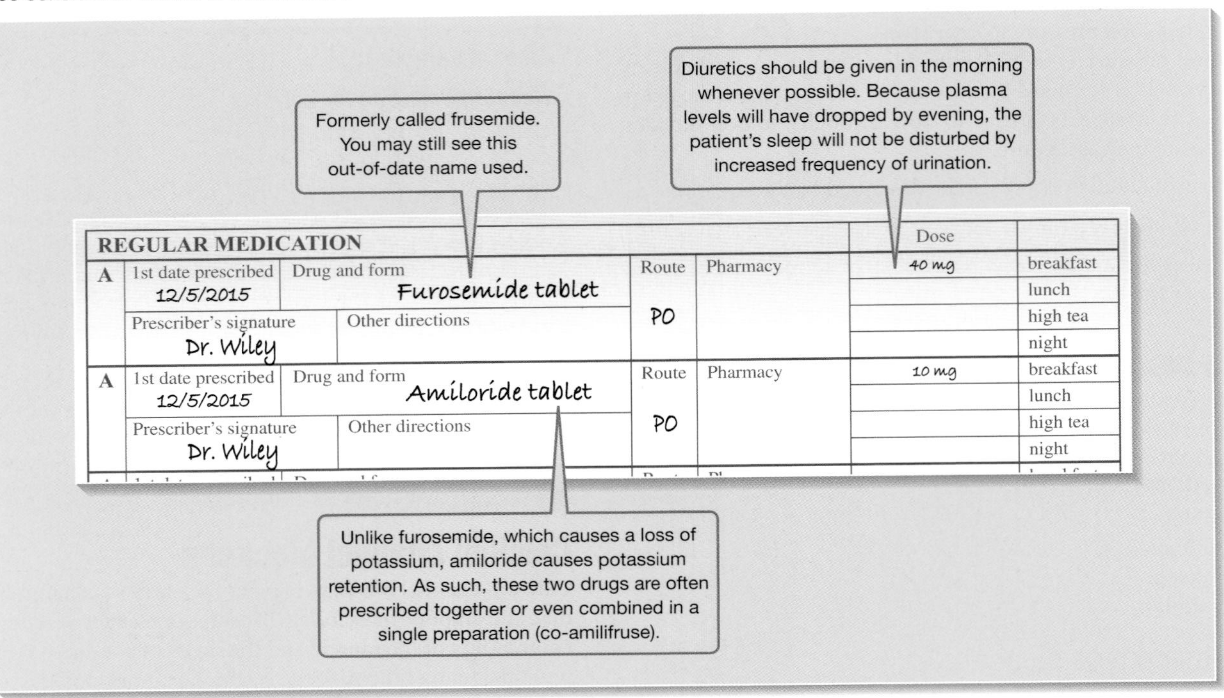


Figure 20.2 The nephron

Figure 20.3 Diuretics block the movement of electrolytes from the tubules into the surrounding blood

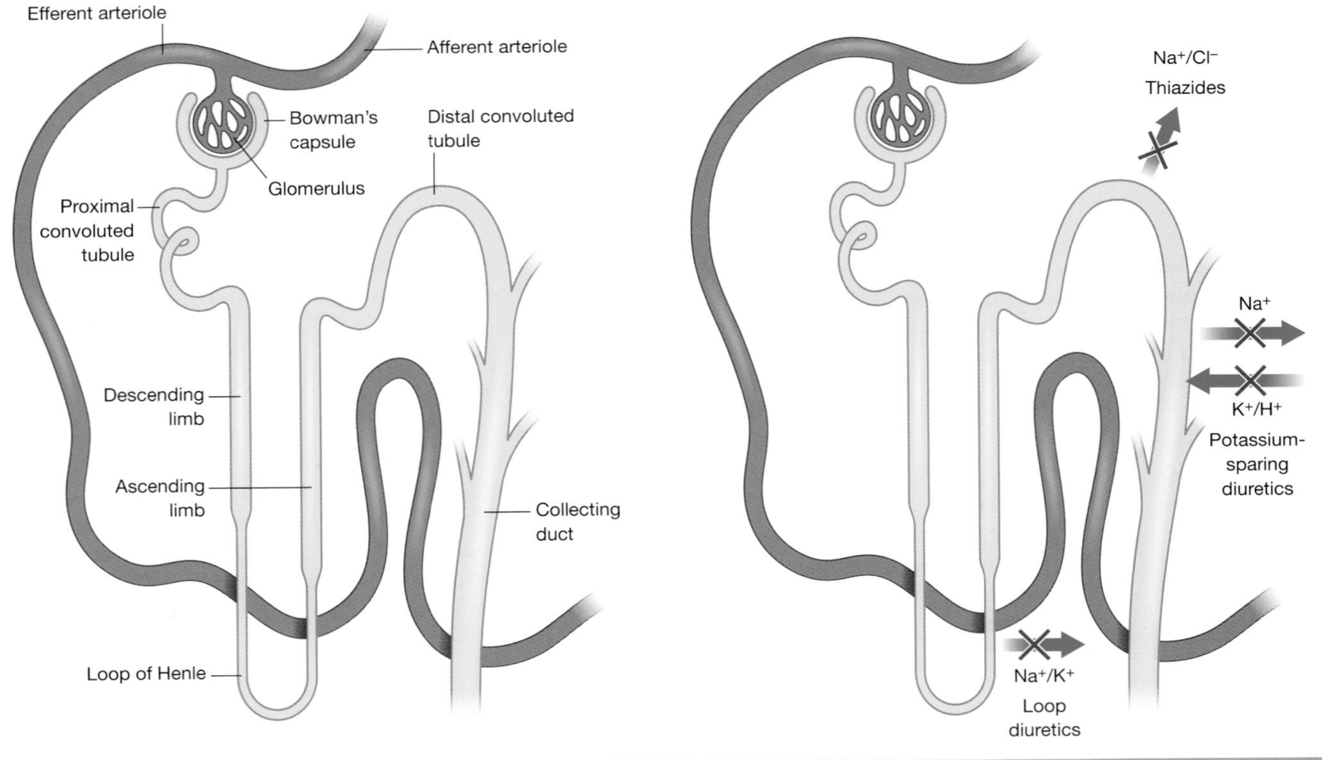

Diuretics are agents that increase urine output with the intention of reducing the volume of fluid in the body. This may be undertaken in situations where the body has become overloaded with fluid, resulting in a range of problems including swelling, heart failure and pulmonary oedema. Diuretics can also be used to lower blood pressure and are often part of a treatment plan for hypertension.

## Pharmacodynamics

As part of the normal production of urine within the nephrons of the kidney (Figure 20.2), electrolytes are transported out of the tubule. This lowers the osmolarity of the fluid within the tubule and raises it in the surrounding blood vessels. Water diffuses from areas of low osmolarity into areas of high osmolarity and therefore approximately 99.5% of the water filtered from the blood in the glomerulus is reabsorbed.

Generally, diuretics block the transport mechanisms that facilitate the movement of the electrolytes from the tubules into the surrounding blood (Figure 20.3). By reducing the difference in osmolarities, less of the water is reabsorbed. Even small reductions in water reabsorption will greatly increase urine output (for example, a reduction of reabsorption of 0.5% from 99.5% to 99% will effectively double the urine output).

There are a range of diuretics available for use. Although they all have the same general effect of increasing urine output, they vary in mechanism of action, inhibiting different transport mechanisms. This means that different diuretics have different effects on the loss and retention of different electrolytes.

Diuretics are generally grouped into the following categories:

- Thiazides.
- Loop diuretics.
- Potassium-sparing diuretics.
- Aldosterone antagonists.
- Osmotic diuretics.

### Thiazides (e.g. bendroflumethiazide)

Thiazides are a commonly used group of diuretics that interfere with the reabsorption of the sodium ions from the distal convoluted tubule. Thiazides are effective in lowering blood pressure but have comparably less effect on blood chemistry than some other diuretics. However, they have been associated with exacerbation of disorders such as gout.

### Loop diuretics (e.g. furosemide)

Loop diuretics reduce the reabsorption of sodium and potassium from the loop of Henle. They are very potent and act very quickly. They can be used to lower blood pressure and reduce fluid retention in chronic treatment, and to stimulate rapid fluid loss in pulmonary oedema. Because loop diuretics reduce the reabsorption of potassium, it is therefore lost from the body resulting in hypokalaemia. This may be addressed by supplementing the patient's potassium intake via intravenous infusion, oral supplements or combining the drug with another agent that will cause potassium retention.

### Potassium-sparing diuretics (e.g. amiloride)

In contrast to loop diuretics, which cause hypokalaemia, potassium-sparing diuretics actually cause potassium retention. Amiloride acts upon the sodium channels in the distal convoluted tubule. Reducing the removal of sodium from the tubule increases its osmolarity and reduces the reabsorption of water, increasing the water content of the urine. By reducing the inflow of sodium into the cell, it indirectly reduces the outflow of potassium.

Potassium-sparing diuretics can increase serum potassium levels and should therefore be used in caution with other agents that might increase potassium levels, such as potassium supplements or angiotensin converting enzyme (ACE) inhibitors. However, the potassium-retaining qualities can be useful to balance out the potassium loss caused by other drugs such as loop diuretics (Figure 20.1). In some cases these drugs are combined in a single formulation (e.g. amiloride and furosemide combined as co-amilofruse).

### Aldosterone antagonists (e.g. spironolactone)

Aldosterone is an endogenous hormone that is part of the body's own control system for maintaining fluid balance, thereby causing an increase in water reabsorption. Aldosterone antagonists block the aldosterone receptor, prevent the increased reabsorption and reduce urine output. Aldosterone antagonists can also contribute to potassium retention.

### Osmotic diuretics (e.g. mannitol)

Administered intravenously, these drugs are solutions of large molecules that dramatically increase the osmolarity of the blood. This causes a net movement of fluid out from the tissues into the blood supply, where it can then be removed by the kidneys. This is a useful method of removing a harmful accumulation of fluid from tissues such as in the relief of cerebral oedema.

### Side effects/adverse drug reactions (ADRs)

#### *Polyuria (excessive passing of urine)*

While this is of course the desired outcome, it can also be problematic. The sudden and urgent need to pass urine can leave patients feeling they cannot go far from a toilet. If mobility is an issue, it can even result in incontinence. This can lead to non-compliance with treatment, or attempts to reduce urine output by drinking less, resulting in dehydration and urinary tract infections.

To try and address this issue, or at least reduce the impact on patients, dosing of diuretics should be scheduled strategically to avoid the need for frequent urination through the night, disrupting sleep.

#### *Postural hypotension (dropping of blood pressure when standing up)*

As the diuretic reduces the circulating volume of the blood, it will cause a drop in blood pressure. This can leave an individual with the symptoms of mild hypotension cold peripheries, dizziness when standing and even fainting.

#### *Hypokaelemia (low potassium)*

As mentioned earlier, some diuretics cause a loss of electrolytes. Loss of potassium can be particularly problematic (a notable side effect of furosemide). Hypokaeleamia can lead to muscle weakness, cramps, cardiac arrhythmias and ectopic heartbeats.

### Other diuretics

There are a variety of other diuretics used to facilitate fluid loss. Information about these less commonly used drugs can be found in the British National Formulary (BNF).

# 21 Respiratory conditions I

**Figure 21.1** An entry from an in-patient medication chart illustrating how salbutamol may be prescribed and some key features to be considered when it is administered

The 100 micrograms listed here denotes the quantity of drug that is supplied with each puff.

A pressurised **metered dose inhaler** (pMDI) should be shaken before each puff.

| REGULAR MEDICATION | | | | | Dose | |
|---|---|---|---|---|---|---|
| A | 1st date prescribed 12/5/2015 | Drug and form Salbutamol 100 micrograms | Route | Pharmacy | 2 puffs | breakfast |
| | | | PO | | | lunch |
| | Prescriber's signature Dr. Wiley | Other directions Use via pMDI- spacer | | | | high tea |
| | | | | | | night |

A pMDI delivers a set quantity of drug with each spray. Using a spacer is the best way to ensure that as much of the drug as possible reaches the lungs.

The term 'respiratory drugs' refers to any drug that affects or is intended to treat the respiratory system. These drugs are often administered by inhalation, although this is not always the case.

Respiratory disease is common throughout the population and particularly in elderly people. It may be a naturally occurring disease, such as asthma, or the result of exposure to toxic or harmful substances (such as cigarette smoke or coal dust). This chapter will focus on the drugs used to treat these types of chronic respiratory conditions.

The British National Formulary (BNF) groups respiratory drugs by their mechanism of action. However, you may also hear them grouped into two categories: **relievers** and **preventers**, especially when used for asthma.

Relievers do not treat the disease: they treat the symptoms. The drug is known as a 'reliever' because it relieves symptoms. Relievers are often only prescribed PRN (as required) when symptoms develop.

Preventers treat the underlying disease. Taken regularly, even in the absence of symptoms, they are intended to prevent future attacks or deterioration of the condition.

## Bronchodilators

These are agents that facilitate the widening of the small airways of the lung, allowing air to flow more easily to and from the alveoli.

## Adrenoceptor agonists

### Common examples

- Salbutamol (Ventolin®).
- Terbutaline.

Salbutamol is probably one of the most commonly used respiratory drugs, often seen in its characteristic blue inhaler and packaging (Figure 21.1).

### Pharmacodynamics

The sympathetic nervous system (SNS) modulates physiological processes by releasing adrenaline into the body. Adrenaline stimulates the production of cyclic adenosine monophosphate (cAMP), which precipitates the relaxation of the smooth muscle in the wall of the bronchiole.

Salbutamol is a beta$_2$ adrenergic agonist. This means that it stimulates the same receptors in the lungs that adrenaline stimulates, and therefore causes bronchodilation.

### Pharmacokinetics

Although commonly administered in some form of inhaler, salbutamol can also be seen to be administered by nebuliser or other routes in a hospital environment. It is fast acting, allowing it to be used to relieve the symptoms of acute attacks.

### Side effects/adverse drug reactions (ADRs)

Because salbutamol stimulates the same receptors as adrenaline, it is unsurprising that the side effects are similar – for example, tachycardia and tremor.

## Antimuscarinic bronchodilators

### Common example

- Ipratropium (Atrovent®).

This is another common respiratory drug, often seen in green packaging.

*Medicines Management for Nurses at a Glance.* First Edition. Simon Young and Ben Pitcher.  Published 2016 by John Wiley & Sons, Ltd.
www.ataglanceseries.com/nursing/medicinesmanagement

### Pharmacodynamics

The parasympathetic nervous system modulates physiological processes using the neurotransmitter acetylcholine (ACh). ACh causes the bronchioles to constrict and obstruct the flow of air into the lungs. Ipratropium is an ACh antagonist, blocking the receptors that the ACh binds to and preventing the constriction of the bronchioles.

Ipratropium is often given in combination with salbutamol because their actions are complementary. There are some preparations that have the two drugs mixed together.

### Pharmacokinetics

Ipratropium is predominantly used in hospitals and administered by nebuliser, although it is also available as an inhaler.

## Theophylline and aminophylline

Theophylline and aminophylline are part of a group of chemicals called xanthines (of which caffeine is also a member). They are used for the treatment of chronic respiratory disease.

### Pharmacodynamics

As discussed earlier in relation to salbutamol, increasing levels of cAMP within the bronchiole walls cause bronchodilation via the relaxation of the smooth muscle. Normally, in order to 'switch off' the bronchodilation, cAMP is converted to inactive 5-adenosine monophosphate (5-AMP). Theophylline inhibits this conversion thereby elevating the levels of cAMP and preventing the bronchodilation from being switched off. This prolongs and enhances the bronchodilation.

### Pharmacokinetics

Unlike most other respiratory drugs, theophylline is not administered by inhalation: it is only administered orally or as an intravenous (IV) infusion.

### Side effects/ADRs

The molecular structure of theophylline is very similar to caffeine. As such, it is unsurprising that many of its side effects are similar to those of caffeine:

- Tachycardia.
- Central nervous system (CNS) stimulation.
- Insomnia.
- Nausea.
- Bad taste in mouth.

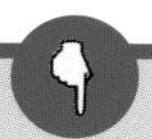

**Clinical pointers**

Theophylline and aminophylline can be toxic. As such, blood tests must be taken to monitor plasma concentration. Prescribing should be brand specific (and only the prescribed brand should be administered) because differences from brand to brand can cause significant fluctuations in plasma concentration.

## Inhaled corticosteroids

- Beclometasone dipropionate.
- Budesonide.
- Fluticasone propionate.
- Mometasone furoate.

### Indications

Corticosteroids have a wide range of effects. One of them is the inhibitory effect that they have on the inflammatory pathway. Some respiratory diseases (including asthma) involve inflammation of the airways. This inflammation narrows the airways and obstructs the flow of air; therefore, reducing the inflammation makes breathing easier. While corticosteroids are commonly given in low doses via inhaler, serious exacerbations of asthma or other respiratory diseases may be treated with much larger oral or IV doses.

### Pharmacodynamics

Corticosteroids stimulate the production of lipocortin-1. This suppresses phospholipase-A2, which blocks the production of inflammatory mediators. The effect of this is to reduce the inflammation of the airways.

### Side effects/ADRs

Corticosteroids are potent drugs that can have many notable side effects. However, the inhaled dose is very small and insignificant compared with the dose of steroids that may be required should the condition deteriorate as a result of not taking a preventer drug.

Steroids are immunosuppressant and patients can therefore develop oral yeast infections.

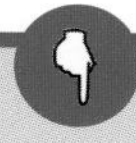

**Clinical pointers**

Corticosteroids are considered preventers and should be administered regularly to prevent exacerbations or asthma attacks. It is important that the patient continues to take the medication even if they feel asymptomatic.

## Leukotriene receptor antagonists

### Common example

- Montelukast.

### Indications

Leukotriene receptor antagonists are 'preventer' drugs intended to prevent the development of symptoms rather than provide immediate relief. They are an option if the more traditional combination of bronchodilators and inhaled corticosteroids has been ineffective.

### Pharmacodynamics

Leukotrienes are inflammatory mediators particularly associated with the respiratory system. They bind to a receptor in the tissues of the lung and enhance inflammation. Leukotriene receptor antagonists block these receptors, preventing the leukotriene from binding and reducing the inflammatory response.

### Pharmacokinetics

Montelukast is taken orally every day, even if the patient has no symptoms.

### Side effects/ADRs

Leukotriene receptor antagonists have fewer side effects than corticosteroids but can cause an array of side effects including hyperkinesia, restlessness, altered mood and sleep disturbances.

# 22 Respiratory conditions II

**Figure 22.1** An entry from an in-patient medication chart illustrating how antihistamine tablets may be prescribed and some key features to be considered when they are administered

Antihistamines are known to cause drowsiness. This could affect the safety of a person driving or using heavy machinery.

| REGULAR MEDICATION | | | | | Dose | |
|---|---|---|---|---|---|---|
| A | 1st date prescribed 12/5/2015 | Drug and form Chlorphenamine tablets | Route | Pharmacy | 4 mg | breakfast |
| | | | | | 4 mg | lunch |
| | Prescriber's signature Dr. Wiley | Other directions May cause drowsiness | PO | | 4 mg | high tea |
| | | | | | 4 mg | night |

Cetirizine is part of a group of non-drowsy antihistamines. They are less lipid soluble so do not enter the brain and make the patient sleepy. However, this slows their entry into the tissues as well, giving them a slower onset of action.

| REGULAR MEDICATION | | | | | Dose | |
|---|---|---|---|---|---|---|
| A | 1st date prescribed 12/5/2015 | Drug and form Cetirizine tablets | Route | Pharmacy | 10 mg | breakfast |
| | | | | | | lunch |
| | Prescriber's signature Dr. Wiley | Other directions | PO | | | high tea |
| | | | | | | night |

In Chapter 21 we looked at drugs that were used to treat more serious chronic respiratory disorders such as asthma and chronic obstructive pulmonary disease (COPD). In this chapter we will look at drugs used for treating other respiratory conditions such as coughs, colds and rhinitis (often induced by allergy).

## Decongestants

- Pseudoephedrine hydrochloride.

### Indications

When a patient has an upper respiratory tract infection, the mucous membranes of the nose can produce large amounts of mucous. This can be unpleasant and inconvenient. Decongestants aim to reduce the amount of mucous produced.

### Pharmacodynamics

Pseudoephedrine is an analogue of adrenaline (epinephrine) and mimics some of its effects. Among a range of actions, it causes vasoconstriction of the small blood vessels that supply the mucous membranes. This reduces the supply of blood, water and nutrients available. Without these raw materials, the mucous membranes produce less mucous.

### Pharmacokinetics

Decongestants can be taken orally as tablets or applied topically using a nasal spray or drops.

### Side effects/adverse drug reactions (ADRs)

Many of the side effects of pseudoephedrine derive from its similarity to adrenaline; these include hypertension, tachycardia, headache, anxiety and restlessness. There have also been reports of urinary retention, which has led to its being used as a 'modern folk remedy' for urinary incontinence; however, this is not a recognised use of this drug.

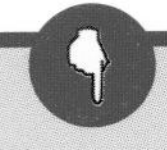

**Clinical pointers**

Pseudoephedrine is a prescription-only medication, but it can be sold to the public in limited amounts. It has notable interactions with some antidepressants (monoamine-oxidase inhibitors [MAOIs]).

## Mucolytics

Also called:

- mucokinetic agents
- mucoactive agents
- mucous-controlling agents.

Examples are:

- carbocisteine
- erdosteine
- mecysteine hydrochloride
- hypertonic sodium chloride
- n-acetylcysteine.

### Indications

Secretions can build up in the lung as a result of inflammation or infection. Mucolytics are designed to help loosen these secretions so that they can be expectorated. If they are not cleared, the patient is at risk of secondary infections or obstruction of the bronchioles (preventing the entry of air into part of the lung).

### Pharmacodynamics

Mucolytics reduce sputum viscosity by splitting the bonds that hold the proteins within the mucous together. As the bonds break, the proteins can move past each other more easily, becoming more fluid and easier to cough up.

### Pharmacokinetics

Mucolytics are most commonly seen as oral syrups, although occasionally the active ingredient is nebulised to get it deep into the lung.

## Antihistamines

### Common examples

- Chlorphenamine (Piriton®).
- Loratadine.
- Cetirizine.

Histamine is a signalling molecule used in a variety of roles throughout the body. One of its key roles is as an inflammatory mediator when it causes the swelling and itching associated with allergic reactions. As their name suggests, antihistamines block the action of histamine. This is useful for treating all forms of allergic reaction but it is commonly used to treat allergic rhinitis (e.g. hay fever, Figure 22.1).

### Pharmacodynamics

Histamine triggers its actions by binding to and activating histamine receptors. Antihistamines block these receptors, thereby preventing the histamine from binding and the receptors from activating.

### Pharmacokinetics and side effects

Because histamine has a variety of roles within the body, blocking histamine receptors can have an equally broad range of side effects. Some of these (particularly drowsiness) are caused by a blockade of the histamine receptors in the brain. As discussed in Chapter 6, for drugs to enter the brain they must be lipid soluble. The older antihistamines are lipid soluble and therefore enter the brain and cause drowsiness. The newer antihistamines are less lipid soluble and therefore do not enter the brain and do not cause drowsiness. As a result, antihistamines are grouped according to whether they are **sedating** or **non-sedating**.

Chlorphenamine (Piriton®) is probably the most well-known sedating antihistamine. Loratadine and cetirizine are commonly used non-sedating antihistamines.

## Oxygen

The importance of oxygen is obvious, but it is not always appreciated that it should be considered a drug.

### Pharmacokinetics

Oxygen is obviously delivered by inhalation; however, there are many types of delivery equipment. Oxygen dosing is set by controlling the rate of flow (measured in litres per minute [L/min]) through the delivery equipment. Changing the flow rate will affect the percentage of the inspired air that will be oxygen. This is referred to as the '$FiO_2$'. It is important to remember that different equipment will provide a different $FiO_2$ at the same flow rate.

### Side effects/ADRs

It might seem unlikely but it is possible to overdose patients with oxygen. In healthy patients, the respiratory rate is controlled by levels of carbon dioxide ($CO_2$) in the blood. However, patients with type 2 respiratory failure are desensitised to $CO_2$ because of the continually elevated levels in their blood. In these patients, breathing is triggered by dropping levels of $O_2$ instead. If you provide a patient with type 2 respiratory failure with too much oxygen, they will not have to breathe very often to maintain adequate levels of $O_2$ and so their respiratory rate will drop. This reduced respiratory rate may be too low to adequately remove the $CO_2$. Because they are desensitised, they will not be aware of the rising levels of $CO_2$ until they become dangerously hypercapnic. However, this should not prevent the use of oxygen in seriously hypoxic patients.

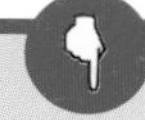

#### Clinical pointers

Oxygen is a drug but it is not classified as a prescription-only medication (POM). This means that technically it does not have to be prescribed in order to be given to a patient. However, within most care environments all drugs are required to be prescribed before they can be administered. In an emergency situation, when the need for supplementary oxygen is urgent and required without delay, it is reasonable to start a patient on oxygen without waiting to get it prescribed. However, this should be immediately reported to a doctor or senior practitioner.

# 23 Opioid analgesics

**Figure 23.1** An entry from an in-patient medication chart illustrating how an opioid analgesic and an opioid antagonist may might be prescribed and some key features to be considered when they are administered

Morphine can be administered in a variety of formulations, including modified-release preparations.

| REGULAR MEDICATION | | | | | Dose | |
|---|---|---|---|---|---|---|
| A | 1st date prescribed 12/5/2015 | Drug and form MST tablets | Route PO | Pharmacy | 5 mg | breakfast |
| | | | | | | lunch |
| | Prescriber's signature Dr. Wiley | Other directions Monitor respiratory rate | | | 5 mg | high tea |
| | | | | | | night |

Morphine can cause respiratory depression. It is important to closely monitor patients who are initiating morphine therapy or who are being given an increased or fast-acting dose.

| AS REQUIRED MEDICATION | | | Maximum is **total** dose per 24 hours including regular medication | | | Cancellation |
|---|---|---|---|---|---|---|
| L | Drug and form Naloxone - Minijet | | Indication Opioid overdose | Prescriber's signature Dr. Wiley | | Date / Time / Dose / Sign — Sign & date |
| | Dose 400 micrograms | Frequency | Maximum | Route IV | Date 12/5/2015 | Pharmacy | Date / Time / Dose / Sign |

If a patient is given too much opioid or is especially sensitive, the drug's action can be reversed using naloxone.

Naloxone is not always charted and may form part of a clinical area's emergency drugs policy.

*Medicines Management for Nurses at a Glance.* First Edition. Simon Young and Ben Pitcher. © 2016 John Wiley & Sons, Ltd. Published 2016 by John Wiley & Sons, Ltd.
www.ataglanceseries.com/nursing/medicinesmanagement

Although pain serves an important role in alerting us to harm and preventing us from continuing to damage ourselves, it is also obviously unpleasant. Throughout the history of civilisation, we have striven to find ways to reduce our experience of pain. Some of the drugs we use are essentially unchanged from those used for hundreds of years; others are newly created synthetic molecules.

## Opioid analgesics

Opioid analgesics refer to drugs that are either derived from opium or are synthetically created molecules that have a similar mechanism of action (Figure 23.1).

### Indications

There are a range of opioids used for a variety of clinical situations. Stronger opioids (e.g. morphine, diamorphine) can be used to control severe pain in palliative care or in post-operative patients. Weaker opioids (codeine) can be used to treat mild to moderate pain.

### Pharmacodynamics

Opioid analgesics stimulate the body's own endogenous analgesic system. When we are hurt, afferent nerve fibres conveying information about pain carry a signal up the spinal cord and into the brain where we experience the sensation of pain. In response, efferent pathways are activated sending nervous impulses from the brain back into the spinal cord. There the nerve fibres release endorphins that bind to receptors on the afferent fibres, preventing them from conducting the sensory information to the brain and thereby reducing the experience of pain. Endorphins are generally only released for a short period of time to allow an injured individual to extricate themselves from a dangerous situation without being crippled by pain.

Opioid analgesics act by binding to the receptors that would normally be bound to by endorphins. Using external agents, we can flood these receptors to create a greater and longer-lasting analgesic effect. Because these receptors were first identified by the action that opioids had on them, they are referred to as 'opioid receptors'.

### Side effects/adverse drug reactions (ADRs)

Opioid analgesic drugs generally share the same range of side effects, the severity of which is generally proportionate to the strength of the opioid. Notable side effects include respiratory depression, nausea and vomiting, constipation, itching of the skin, drowsiness, confusion and dependence.

## Commonly used opioid analgesics

### Strong opioids

**Morphine** is one of the most common and important opioid analgesics. It is the 'gold standard' when discussing analgesics (i.e. the effectiveness of other agents is often discussed in terms of how they compare with morphine). Morphine can be delivered intravenously and is often used for the control of post-operative pain. It can also be administered orally in tablet or even syrup form, when it can be used for the treatment of pain in chronic conditions or in palliative care.

Morphine's effectiveness as an analgesic is matched by the strength of its side effects. Many patients experience nausea, vomiting and constipation. Because of the potential for respiratory depression, the patient's respiratory rate should be monitored.

**Diamorphine** (often referred to as 'heroin') is molecularly similar to morphine but with two acetyl groups added, which prevent the molecule from binding to the opioid receptor. This means that diamorphine is actually a prodrug that must be metabolised by the body to convert it to the active agent. If diamorphine is administered orally, the acetyl groups are removed by the liver in first-pass metabolism and it converts to morphine. However, if the drug is administered via a parenteral route, it remains acetylated. This makes it much more lipid soluble, which allows it to enter the brain far more easily. Once in the brain, the diamorphine is metabolised back to morphine to allow it to take effect. The greater lipid solubility of the diamorphine allows it to be effective at lower doses.

**Alfentanil** and **remifentanil** can be used intravenously for analgesia during surgery or while a patient is being cared for in critical care. Their short half-life allows the level of analgesia to be tightly controlled.

**Fentanyl** can be used for intra-operative pain control but also administered by a transdermal patch. This is an effective way of supplying a consistent dose over a long period of time.

**Methadone**, while more widely known for its use in the treatment of opioid addiction, is in itself an effective analgesic. It has a longer half-life than morphine and therefore requires less frequent dosing.

**Pethidine** is most well known for its use as an analgesic in labour. It is less effective than morphine but also has milder side effects (particularly constipation).

**Tramadol** can be administered orally or intravenously and is a moderate-strength analgesic that can be used to treat pain in chronic or acute conditions. While it is primarily considered an opioid analgesic, it has an additional mechanism of action in which it modulates the release of noradrenaline and serotonin (5-HT), further reducing the conduction of painful stimuli to the brain. Perhaps because of this dual action, it is able to deliver effective pain control with fewer side effects.

### Weak opioids

**Codeine** is usually delivered orally via tablet or as a linctus. It is most commonly seen combined with paracetamol in a single tablet (co-codamol). Because codeine is generally a weaker analgesic, it also usually has less dangerous side effects. However, concerns have been raised about its potential for dependence and it is known as one of the most constipating of the opioid analgesics.

**Dihydrocodeine** is similar to codeine although more potent at higher doses. It is accompanied by more severe side effects.

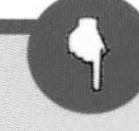

**Clinical pointers**

Opioids can be potentially lethal in overdose. The drug **naloxone** is a competitive antagonist for opioid receptors. When administered, it displaces the opioid analgesic from the receptors and prevents it from binding again. This essentially reverses the action of the opioid, immediately removing the respiratory depression, sedation and analgesic actions of the drug.

# 24 Anxiolytics and hypnotics

Figure 24.1 An entry from an in-patient medication chart illustrating how zopiclone may be prescribed and some key features to be considered when it is administered

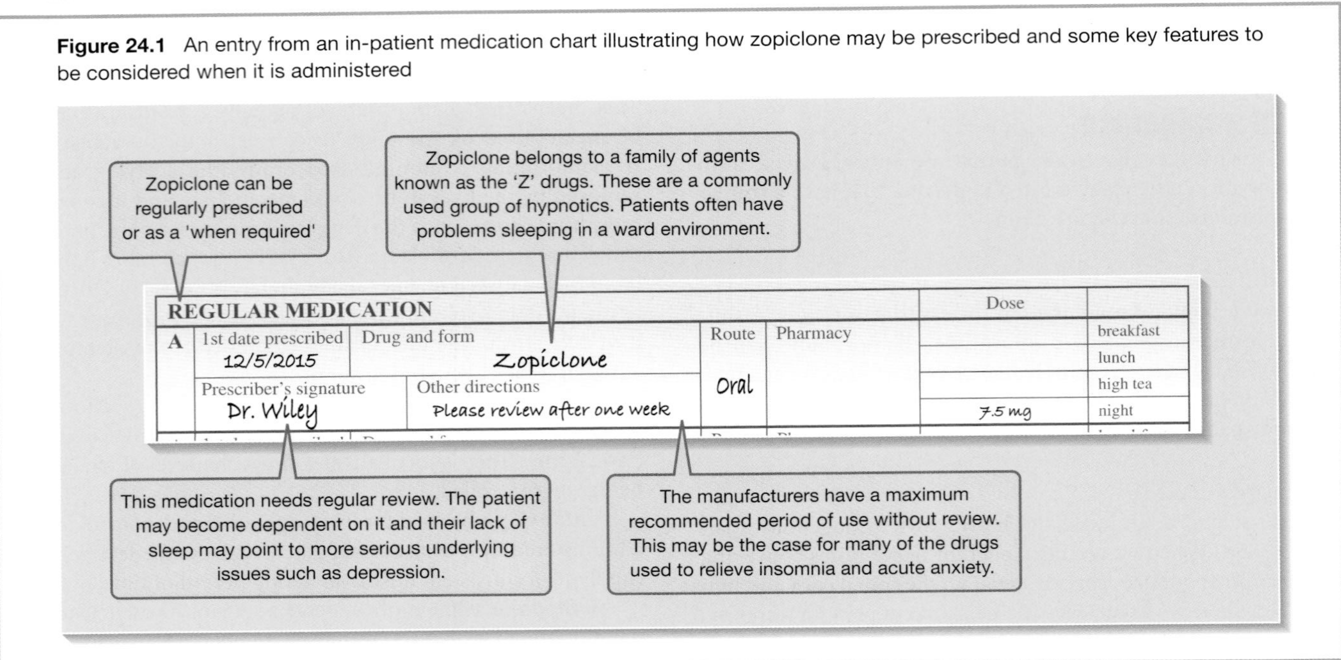


Anxiolytics are medicines that are used to treat the symptoms of the various classes of anxiety disorder, such as generalised anxiety disorder (GAD), social phobias and panic disorders. Anxiety is a symptom associated with several mental health disorders including depression and substance misuse.

Hypnotics are medications that are designed to assist a patient in getting to sleep (Figure 24.1). Defining the parameters of a normal sleep pattern is very difficult because the amount of sleep patients need varies. Insomnia is one of the defining symptoms in diagnosing depression and is a medical disorder in its own right.

## Benzodiazepines

- Diazepam.

The benzodiazepines are a group of drugs that are used as both anxiolytics and hypnotics. They should be prescribed at the lowest doses possible and for the shortest possible duration because they are associated with dependence. Diazepam has a relatively quick action and is used to treat anxiety for short periods. Other benzodiazepines, such as nitrazepam and temazepam, are typically used as hypnotics.

### Pharmacokinetics and pharmacodynamics

When used to treat anxiety, benzodiazepines are given orally. Occasionally they are dosed parenterally or via the rectal route. Diazepam has a peak plasma concentration 60–90 minutes after oral dosing and has a long half-life (the drug and its active metabolites persist in the body for a long period of time). The drug is lipid soluble and readily crosses the blood–brain barrier. It is typically dosed two to three times daily for anxiety.

The benzodiazepines are functional gamma amino butyric acid (GABA) agonists. They work by increasing the efficiency of the natural brain chemical, GABA. This in turn decreases the excitability of neurons, which reduces the communication between neurons and exerts a calming 'inhibitory' effect on many the functions of the brain.

### Notable contra-indications/cautions and warnings

All benzodiazepines can cause drowsiness, and that drowsiness may persist in some patients. This can affect or influence skilled tasks such as driving. Alcohol potentiates this effect. Respiratory disease and respiratory depression are cautions/contra-indications to benzodiazepine use.

### Side effects/adverse drug reactions (ADRs)

These include drowsiness, light-headedness, confusion and ataxia (particularly in older patients). Dependence on these agents is always a consideration.

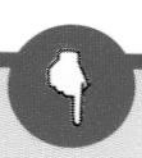

**Clinical pointers**

Diazepam is commonly used to assist with alcohol withdrawal. There is a large variance between the doses used to treat anxiety and those used to treat alcohol withdrawal (Chapter 28).

## Buspirone

### Pharmacokinetics and pharmacodynamics

Buspirone is an oral anxiolytic that acts on a variety of neurotransmitter systems. It does not have the same pharmacodynamics as the benzodiazepines and does not typically cause the same levels of drowsiness. It is dosed two to three times daily. There is a lower dependence and misuse potential with buspirone than with the benzodiazepines.

### Notable contra-indications/cautions and warnings

Buspirone is contra-indicated in epilepsy. The drug can cause drowsiness and has a warning regarding its adverse influence on skilled tasks and driving.

### Side effects/ADRs

Side effects include nausea, headache, dizziness and increased anxiety. Others include dry mouth, tachycardia, palpitations, chest pain, drowsiness, confusion, seizures, fatigue and sweating.

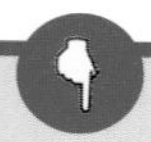

**Clinical pointers**

The drug takes up to 2 weeks to exert its full anxiolytic effect and patients typically report poor efficacy because they associate the quick action and drowsiness of diazepam with an anxiolytic effect.

## Antidepressants and beta-blockers

In addition to the benzodiazepines and buspirone, the selective serotonin re-uptake inhibitors (SSRIs) and the beta-blocker, Propranolol, have been used to treat anxiety. SSRIs such as citalopram, escitalopram, fluoxetine and sertraline are licensed for conditions including obsessive–compulsive disorder, GAD and panic disorder. Propranolol is used to treat the non-psychological symptoms of anxiety such as tremor and palpitations. It is not effective in directly relieving worry and fear but relieving physical symptoms may assist with psychological symptoms.

## Hypnotics – the 'Z' drugs (Zaleplon, Zopiclone and Zolpidem)

The 'Z' drugs are hypnotics that are not members of the benzodiazepine chemical family. As with all hypnotics, they are designed for short-term use. Dependence can occur with this group of agents.

### Pharmacokinetics and pharmacodynamics

The Z drugs are dosed orally; they are administered at night prior to the timing of sleep onset and act by influencing GABA transmission in the central nervous system.

### Notable contra-indications/cautions and warnings

Zopiclone is contra-indicated in patients with myasthenia gravis, respiratory failure, severe sleep apnoea syndrome and severe hepatic insufficiency.

### Side effects/ADRs

Taste disturbance is often associated with these drugs. Other side effects such as nausea and gastro-intestinal distress, dizziness, drowsiness and dry mouth may also occur. Paradoxical effects such as insomnia and sleep walking are rare ADRs.

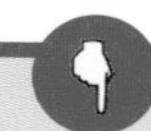

**Clinical pointers**

Benzodiazepines such as temazepam, nitrazepam and lormetazepam are typically used as hypnotics. These drugs have intermediate durations of action and their effects may continue into the day following administration. This can be important when caring for a patient in the morning because they may still be under the influence of hypnotics from the previous night. This is commonly termed the 'hangover' effect.

Care must be taken when administering sedating drugs such as the benzodiazepines and the Z drugs. They all cause drowsiness, light-headedness and ataxia. They have been associated with falls in elderly patients, and these can have serious consequences.

In addition to the hypnotics mentioned, sedating antihistamines (such as promethazine), melatonin and chloral derivatives are used as hypnotic agents.

# Antipsychotics

**Figure 25.1** An entry from an in-patient medication chart illustrating how clozapine (an atypical antipsychotic) may be prescribed and some key features to be considered when it is administered

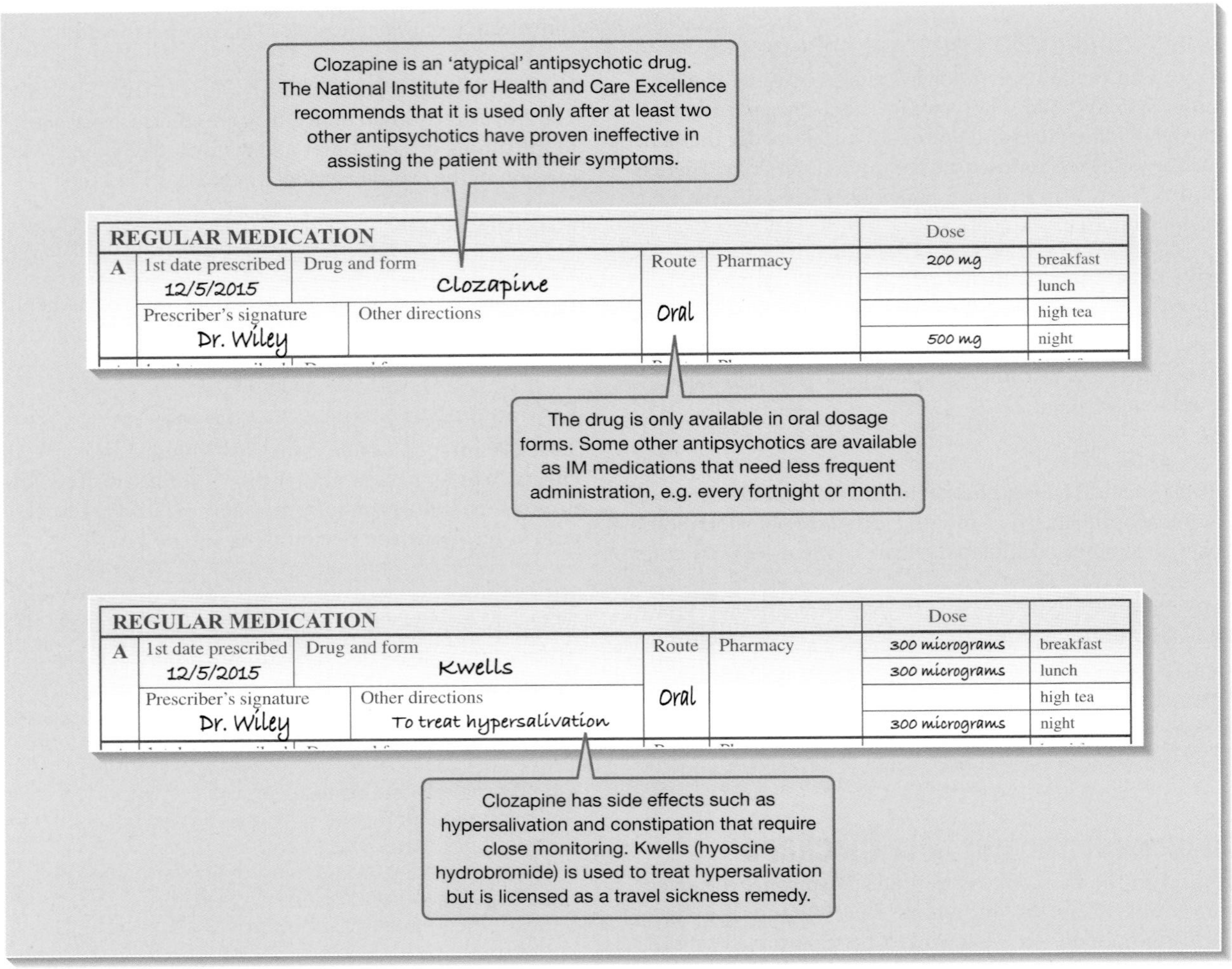

Antipsychotic medication can be used in a variety of mental health conditions (Figure 25.1). Despite being named 'antipsychotics', they are used to treat other conditions such as mania and to 'control' challenging behaviour. In practice, the medications are used for short-term management of acute psychotic episodes in which patients pose harm to themselves or those around them. In the longer term, they are used to control the 'positive' symptoms such as hallucinations and delusions associated with lifelong conditions like schizophrenia. However, they are less effective at managing the 'negative' symptoms such as apathy, social withdrawal and anhedonia.

This group of drugs is sometimes called 'neuroleptics' or 'tranquilizers'. This nomenclature is still used; however, it is outdated and misleading.

## First- and second-generation antipsychotics

The antipsychotics are usually classified as either first or second generation. The first-generation antipsychotics are the oldest (chlorpromazine was the first to be marketed). Drugs that belong to the first generation have similar side-effect profiles and are associated with drowsiness (varying degrees), blurred vision, hypotension and, most importantly, the extrapyramidal side effects (EPSEs) such as akathisia (restlessness), dystonia (abnormal face and body movements), parkinsonian symptoms (symptoms that appear similar to some of those of Parkinson's disease) and tardive dyskinesia (rhythmic, involuntary movements of the face, jaw and tongue). These EPSEs are distressing for the patient, and some may be irreversible and difficult to manage.

The second-generation antipsychotics are generally newer and less associated with EPSEs. Many are better at treating the negative symptoms of schizophrenia. However, they have other side effects that are important to note. They are more frequently associated with cardiovascular side effects and many (e.g. clozapine and olanzapine) are associated with significant weight gain. Some of the second-generation drugs are associated with the development of type II diabetes in patients taking the medications long term. Clozapine is usually reserved for use in treatment-resistant schizophrenia.

Despite the bleak picture of side effects noted earlier, these drugs are effective and truly liberating. The treatment of patients with certain mental health disorders before the introduction of these drugs would, by today's standards, be described as barbaric. The transformation of the care of patients with serious mental health issues, in combination with other effective pharmacological therapies, has enabled patients to be treated in their own home rather than in hospital settings.

### Pharmacokinetics and pharmacodynamics

The antipsychotics are available in a variety of formulations. Preparations such as Clopixol Acuphase® are used as intramuscular (IM) injections for the management of acute psychosis. Short-acting formulations are used in what are commonly termed 'rapid tranquilization' situations when a patient requires acute treatment. Longer-acting preparations of the same drug can be used in the maintenance phase to manage their ongoing symptoms. Some clever formulation work has led to the development of antipsychotics that are administered by IM injections weekly, fortnightly or even monthly. This ensures that the patient has received their medication (an aid to compliance) and also allows the focus of a patient's care to centre around their need, rather than on issues related to medication administration. Examples of longer-acting products include 'depots' such as Piportil depot® and Haldol decanoate®, and long-acting preparations such as Risperdal Consta® and Xeplion®.

There are also a range of oral and orodispersible medications that are designed for ease of administration and compliance (e.g. aripiprazole).

The major role of these drugs is to block the action of dopamine in the brain. They need to act on specific areas of the brain, predominantly the mesolimbic system (associated with reward and desire) and the mesocortical system (associated with cognition, motivation and emotional response). It is hypothesised that an overactivity of dopamine in these systems is responsible for the emergence of the positive and negative symptoms associated with schizophrenia.

### Notable contra-indications/cautions and warnings

The most notable general cautions are associated with cardiovascular disease. Many antipsychotic agents cause electrocardiogram (ECG) changes and are associated with conditions such as QT interval prolongation. Before commencing many antipsychotics, a cardiovascular examination and a baseline ECG are required. Patients with conditions such as schizophrenia require annual physical health checks.

Some antipsychotics cause photosensitisation and warnings to avoid direct sunlight will accompany their use. Many cause drowsiness and are prescribed with warnings regarding driving and consuming alcohol.

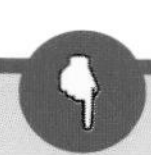

**Clinical pointers**

Many skills are required of a nurse in caring for a patient taking antipsychotics. Being aware of the needs of the patient is primary, as are monitoring for side effects associated with the therapy (e.g. being aware of the signs and symptoms of type II diabetes as well as emergent EPSEs) and understanding the roles that medication plays in managing specific side effects (e.g. hysoscine in managing hypersalivation associated with clozapine).

### Monitoring

Monitoring undertaken while undergoing antipsychotic therapy may involve:

- blood pressure
- pulse
- temperature
- weight/height – body mass index (BMI)
- blood glucose
- ECG
- white cell count and differential blood counts
- cholesterol
- urea and electrolytes
- liver function tests.

Medication such as clozapine requires particular blood monitoring in order to continue therapy. Clozapine has been associated with neutropenia (low blood neutrophil count), which can be fatal if not detected and treated promptly. Clozapine therapy usually requires blood tests to be taken at weekly, fortnightly or monthly intervals, and even for a short period after the discontinuation of therapy.

# 26 Depression

Figure 26.1 Two entries from an in-patient medication chart illustrating how two different antidepressants (one SSRI and one 'tricyclic-related' antidepressant) may be prescribed and some key features to be considered when they are administered

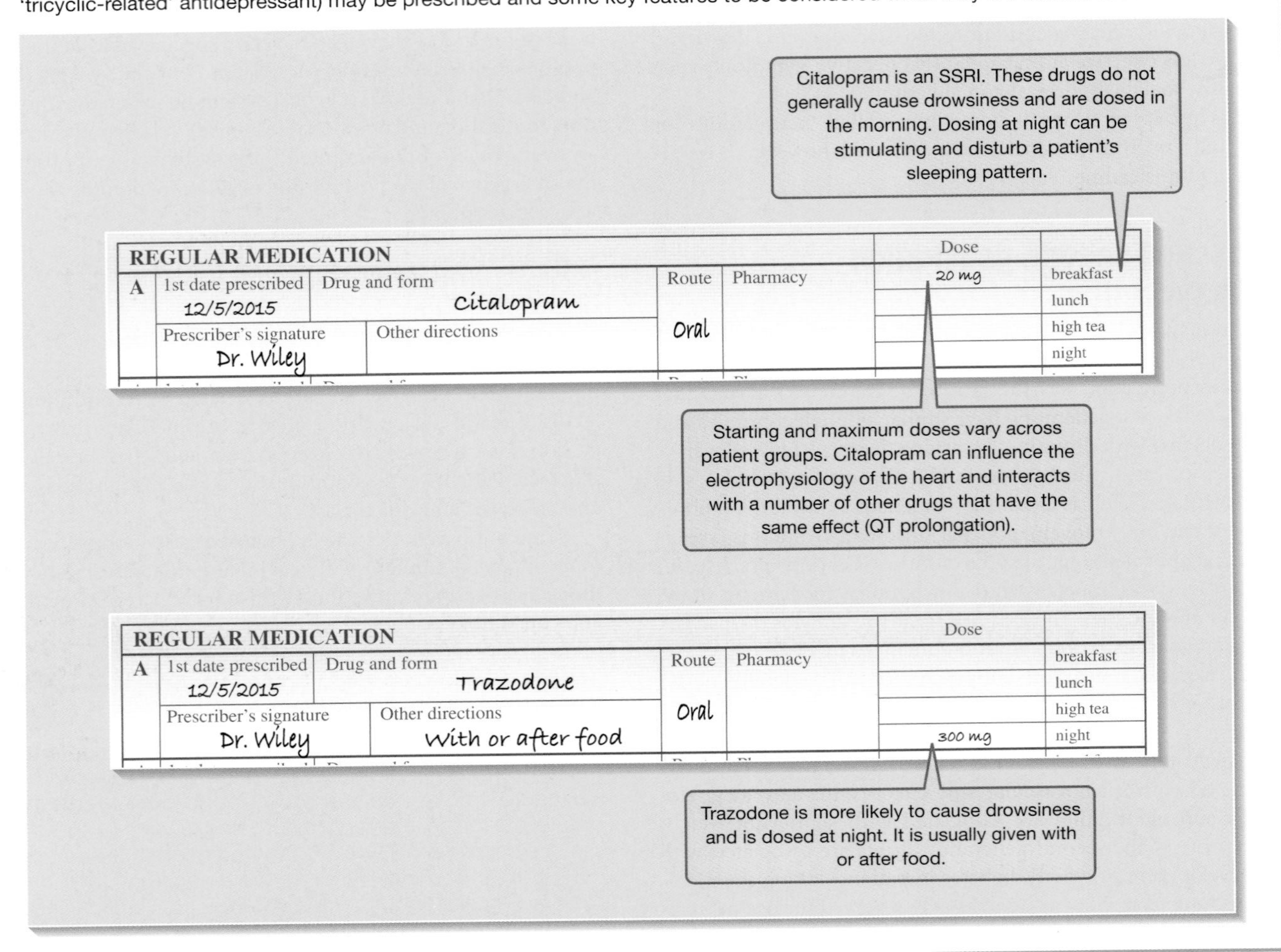


While many people will often feel sad, low or 'depressed', most will have these symptoms for a few days or a couple of weeks, before they pass and the person's mood returns to its normal pattern.

In the case of depression, the feeling of low mood (and accompanying symptoms) persist and develop into a condition that interferes with the quality of that person's life.

A patient suffering with depression might:

- feel unhappy most of the time (but perhaps feel a little better in the evenings)
- lose interest in life and unable to enjoy anything
- find it harder to make decisions
- be less able to cope with things
- feel utterly tired
- feel restless and agitated
- lose their appetite and experience weight loss (or comfort eat and gain weight)
- take 1–2 hours to get off to sleep, and then wake up earlier than usual
- lose interest in sex
- lose self-confidence
- feel useless, inadequate and hopeless
- avoid other people
- feel irritable
- feel worse at a particular time each day, usually in the morning
- think of suicide.

The British National Formulary (BNF) categorises antidepressants into tricyclic and related drugs, monoamine-oxidase inhibitors (MAOIs), selective serotonin re-uptake inhibitors (SSRIs) and others. The most commonly prescribed antidepressants are the SSRIs. These include drugs such as fluoxetine (Prozac®), citalopram (Cipramil®) and sertraline (Lustral®) (Figure 26.1).

## SSRIs

These drugs are so-called because of their pharmacodynamic mechanism of action. They are by far the most frequently encountered in clinical practice. Their side-effect profile is preferential to those of the other drug groups and they are safer in overdose than the other antidepressants. The National Institute for Health and Care Excellence (NICE) suggests they are the most suitable to use, and that the person taking the antidepressant should be involved in choosing their medication.

### Pharmacokinetics and pharmacodynamics

All SSRIs are given orally and some are available in liquid form for those who cannot swallow solid dosage forms. They are usually taken once daily, typically in the morning. Most patients feel more alert when taking this group of drugs so dosing at night is usually not recommended (unless the patient demonstrates idiosyncratic drowsiness). The drugs act by selectively inhibiting the re-uptake of serotonin (5-HT), a neurotransmitter associated with elevated mood.

### Notable contra-indications/cautions and warnings

Cautions include use in patients with epilepsy, cardiac disease, diabetes mellitus and those at risk of bleeding (especially gastrointestinal bleeding). The drugs can impair skilled tasks. They are associated with withdrawal syndromes: patients do not become addicted or dependent but they do experience withdrawal syndromes if the drugs are stopped suddenly. Their use in children and adults under 18 years of age carries a warning in the BNF. The summaries of product characteristics (SPCs) of the individual drugs give further details about their suitability for use in specific subgroups of patients.

### Side effects/adverse drug reactions (ADRs)

The side effects commonly associated with SSRIs include GI and hypersensitivity reactions, and anorexia and weight loss. The drugs cause fewer cardiovascular side effects than the tricyclic antidepressants (TCAs). The SPCs detail their side effects.

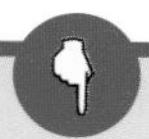

**Clinical pointers**

SSRIs have a wide range of half-lives that may make some more suitable than others for particular patients. Certain SSRIs have undergone limited testing in patients who have suffered cardiovascular problems such as myocardial infarctions (MIs) and strokes. The literature around depression and physical illness has data on the most suitable to use. This area of knowledge is constantly developing.

Some SSRIs are also licensed for other conditions such as bulimia nervosa and obsessive–compulsive disorder.

## Tricyclic and related antidepressants

The tricyclics are the oldest group of synthetic antidepressants. They are so-called because their chemical structure has three 'rings' of carbon atoms – the related drugs have similar properties but different chemical structures.

### Pharmacokinetics and pharmacodynamics

Tricyclics are administered orally. They are used for depression but some are also used to treat conditions such as neuralgia. They act by blocking the re-uptake of serotonin and noradrenaline. Each has a slightly different profile of action. In most patients they can be administered daily because they have long half-lives; occasionally doses will be split, usually to minimise side effects.

### Notable contra-indications/cautions and warnings

Cautions to the use of tricyclics include cardiovascular disease, epilepsy and diabetes. They can cause cardiovascular and epileptogenic effects that are dangerous in overdose. They are contra-indicated post-MI, in arrhythmias and in the manic phase of mood disorders.

### Side effects/ADRs

This group of drugs has prominent antimuscarinic side effects such as drowsiness, dry mouth and constipation.

## Other antidepressants

Medications such as venlafaxine, mirtazapine and duloxetine may have pharmacological profiles that suit the requirements of patients better than the SSRIs and TCAs.

Venlafaxine and duloxetine are serotonin-noradrenaline reuptake inhibitors (SNRIs), a mechanism akin to that of the SSRIs and tricyclics. Mirtazapine is a centrally active presynaptic $\alpha_2$ adrenergic antagonist. The inhibition of the presynaptic $\alpha_2$ adrenergic receptor results in increased central noradrenergic and serotonergic neurotransmission.

MAOIs are less frequently used because of their side-effect profiles and their interaction with foodstuffs.

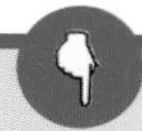

**Clinical pointers**

Antidepressants of all categories take several weeks to work. In observing patients taking them you may see some changes and improvement in their mood within 3–4 weeks but patients will typically take longer to feel different. The exact reason for this is not clearly understood. Using antidepressants is often about understanding a patient's symptoms, patience and careful observation. Changing an antidepressant after 2 weeks of adherent treatment is unwise because this is not enough time to establish whether the therapy is working. Reasons for discontinuing usually centre on side effects that are too troublesome for the patient.

# 27 Epilepsy

**Figure 27.1** An entry from an in-patient medication chart illustrating how phenytoin (Epanutin®) may be prescribed and some key features to be considered when it is administered

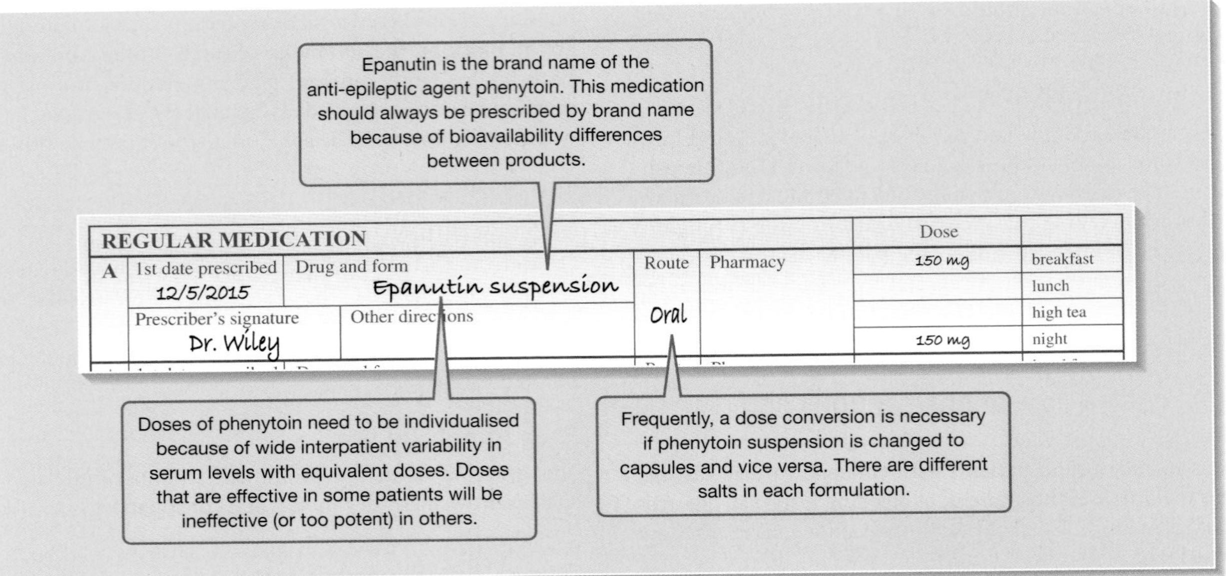


Table 27.1 Table illustrating the CHM categories of anti-epileptic medicines. This outlines the recommendations with regards to swapping between the products of various manufacturers. Examples are illustrative and are not an exhaustive list.

| CHM category | Recommendation | Examples of drug included in the category |
|---|---|---|
| 1 | Patients should be maintained on a specific product from one manufacturer | Carbamazepine, phenobarbital, phenytoin and primidone |
| 2 | The continued supply of one manufacturer's product is based on clinical judgement and pertinent patient history | Clobazam, lamotrigine, topirimate and valproate |
| 3 | It is not usually necessary to ensure that patients receive one particular manufacturer's product unless there are patient concerns e.g. a risk of confusion or anxiety because of manufacturer's differences | Gabapentin, levetiracetam and vigabatrin |

When considering medication used in epilepsy, two perspectives should be considered: medication used to control epilepsies and medication used to treat **status epilepticus**. This section will focus on the drugs used to control epilepsy (Figure 27.1).

The objective of epilepsy treatment is to maintain the patient in a seizure-free state using the lowest dose and number of medications possible. Monotherapy is a primary goal but not always possible. The dose of medication(s) used is often a balance between the dose needed to control seizures and the side effects associated with that medication. The British National Formulary (BNF) lists in excess of 20 agents used to treat the various classifications of epilepsy. This section will focus on two medications that are used in epilepsy for which there are important considerations.

## Anti-epileptic medication

When selecting an anti-epileptic treatment, the cluster of syndromes associated with the diagnosis of epilepsy is considered. However, anti-epileptic medication is often classified as treating a particular type of seizure or classification of seizure. Other important considerations include age, gender (several anti-epileptic medicines have teratogenic effects and may have other effects *in utero*), comorbidities and other medications taken (some anti-epileptic medications are associated with several drug interactions).

## Valproate

### Pharmacokinetics and pharmacodynamics

Valproate is available in tablet, controlled-release tablet, liquid, granules, capsule and parenteral dosage forms. It is used to treat tonic–clonic seizures, particularly in generalised epilepsy. It is a first-line choice in treating generalised tonic–clonic seizures, focal seizures, generalised absences and myoclonic seizures, and it can be used in atypical absence seizures. The medication is typically dosed 1–3 times daily depending on its use and formulation. The purpose of the controlled-release formulations is to reduce the frequency of the dose and the incidence of acute side effects associated with taking a dose. The half-life of valproate (chrono form; 'chrono' is a controlled-release formulation of sodium valproate) is between 8 and 12 hours in duration, but shorter in children. Valproate is believed to potentiate the inhibitory action of gamma amino butyric acid (GABA).

### Notable contra-indications/cautions and warnings

Liver function needs to be monitored before initiating therapy and 6-monthly thereafter. Full blood counts need to be performed regularly too, because valproate is associated with the development of blood dyscrasia. Its use is also associated with pancreatitis. Nurses should be aware of the signs and symptoms of blood dyscrasia, hepatic toxicity and pancreatitis associated with valproate use.

### Side effects/adverse drug reactions (ADRs)

There are many side effects associated with valproate use. Nausea and diarrhoea are often encountered. Hyperammoniaemia and thrombocytopenia are also notable. Because the drug acts centrally, it can also interfere with mood (irritability and anxiety) and with alertness.

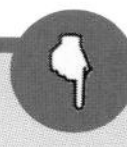

**Clinical pointers**

- The BNF and summary of product characteristics (SPC) give detailed information about the use of valproate in breastfeeding, pregnancy and liver disease.
- The drug is involved in several interactions with other drugs.
- Sodium valproate, semisodium valproate and valproic acid are different chemical variants of valproate. Take care when administering valproate preparations because they will have different doses and indications.
- Valproate is also used to treat bipolar disorder/mood disorders, and to a lesser extent to prevent migraine.

## Carbamazepine

### Pharmacokinetics and pharmacodynamics

Carbamazepine is available as tablets (including modified-release and chewable tablets), liquid and suppositories. It is the drug of choice for simple and complex focal seizures and a first-line treatment option for generalised tonic–clonic seizures. Carbamazepine is also used as adjunctive treatment for focal seizures when monotherapy has been ineffective.

### Notable contra-indications/cautions and warnings/side effects/ADRs

There are significant cautions and contra-indications associated with carbamazepine use – blood, hepatic and skin disorders among them.

The most common side effects include dry mouth, nausea and vomiting. Others include oedema, ataxia, dizziness, drowsiness, fatigue, headache, hyponatraemia and blood disorders.

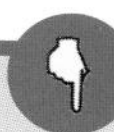

**Clinical pointers**

Carbamazepine therapy should be initiated at a low dose and built up slowly with increments of 100–200 mg every 2 weeks. The drug is also used in trigeminal neuralgia, neuropathy, prevention of seizures associated with alcohol withdrawal and in mood disorders.
It is important that controlled-release tablets are swallowed whole and not chewed or broken (unless the manufacturer specifies that this can be done).

## General advice

The BNF has guidelines on stopping and swapping anti-epileptic agents. As with any drugs, swapping from one product to another has its own set of risks. Abrupt withdrawal of anti-epileptic medication is inadvisable unless continuing the therapy poses a risk to the patient.

In 2013, the Medicines and Healthcare Products Regulatory Agency (MHRA) issued a press release and guidance on the use of anti-epileptics. A review was undertaken by the Commission on Human Medicines (CHM), which explored the issue of patients taking (or being administered/dispensed) the same anti-epileptic drugs manufactured by different pharmaceutical companies. They concluded there was no evidence of harm in using different brands of generic medicines but there was the possibility of the loss of seizure control and differences in side effects if drugs made by different generic manufacturers were continually being changed.

The CHM placed the drugs into three categories as shown in Table 27.1.

# Alcohol: detoxification

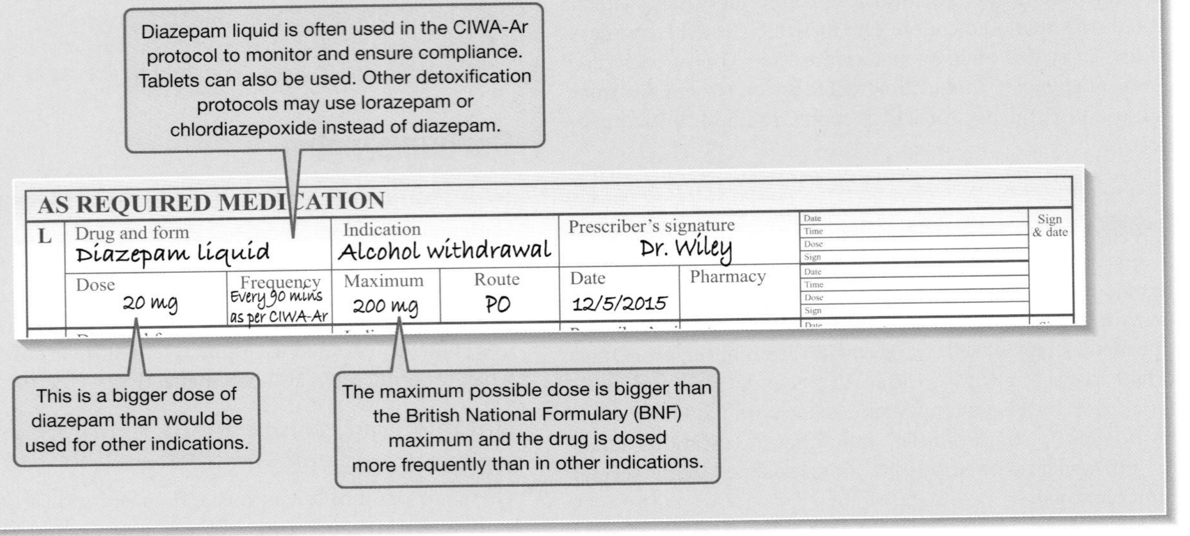


**Figure 28.1** An entry from an in-patient medication chart illustrating how diazepam in the context of CIWA-Ar may be prescribed and some key features to be considered when it is administered

Alcohol is one of the most commonly consumed recreational psychoactive substances in the UK. While many people enjoy alcohol with little or no consequence to their health, some drink an amount that is harmful to themselves and to those around them. Ongoing harmful and hazardous drinking patterns and the ill health related to excessive alcohol intake cost the NHS £21 billion per year.

There are many psychosocial interventions that are used to assist those who misuse alcohol. These include counselling, specific therapies (cognitive behavioural therapy and group therapies such as those offered by Alcoholics Anonymous) and legal and financial support. Alongside these interventions, medication management in alcohol misuse falls broadly into two categories:

1 Medication used in the detoxification process.

2 Medication used to maintain abstinence from drinking alcohol.

## Medication that aids in the detoxification process

Alcohol is termed a central nervous system (CNS) depressant. This essentially means that is suppresses many of the functions of the CNS by facilitating the action of the inhibitory neurotransmitter, gamma amino butyric acid (GABA). It causes drowsiness and impairs motor control and cognitive function. If an alcohol-dependent patient stops drinking alcohol suddenly (e.g. to undertake their own 'detox'), this leaves their brain without the constant depressant effect of the alcohol. The usual response of the brain in this circumstance is to release excitatory neurotransmitters (which have been suppressed for a long period of time); this often results in a neurotoxic effect and may even cause permanent, irreversible brain damage.

When patients undergo detoxification in a community setting (e.g. at home) or as an inpatient, the benzodiazepine, diazepam, is used to aid the process (Figure 28.1). Alcohol and diazepam have a 'cross tolerance' and the diazepam can be administered to pharmacologically substitute for the alcohol that is leaving the patient's body. The diazepam is frequently administered as the symptoms of the withdrawal dictate. This is termed a 'symptom-triggered' detoxification process whereby the diazepam is administered at fixed intervals depending on the withdrawal symptoms (and their intensity) that are being experienced by the patient. The most commonly used symptom-triggered scale is the Clinical Institute Withdrawal Assessment of Alcohol Scale, Revised (CIWA-Ar).

### Posology, pharmacokinetics and pharmacodynamics

When used as part of the CIWA-Ar, the benzodiazepines are given orally as tablets or sometimes as liquid. The patient is assessed using the scale at the beginning of the detoxification and every 90 minutes subsequently. If the symptom score is 11 or more, then 20 mg of diazepam are administered. This continues until the symptoms of withdrawal subside (the duration of treatment varies but is often less than 24 hours). The usual daily maximum of diazepam is 200 mg (although this dose is rarely administered). All withdrawal regimes have key signposted points that require a doctor to be called.

Like alcohol, the benzodiazepines are functional GABA agonists. Benzodiazepines work by increasing the efficiency of the natural brain chemical, GABA, which in turn decreases the excitability of neurons. This reduces the communication between neurons and exerts a calming 'braking' effect on many of the functions of the brain. This similarity in action allows the benzodiazepine to be used to suppress the unpleasant side effects of withdrawal.

### Side effects/adverse drug reactions (ADRs)

These include drowsiness, light-headedness, confusion and ataxia (particularly in older patients). They are often difficult to distinguish from the effects of alcohol and the withdrawal process. The tendency for dependence on diazepam to develop during detoxification is unlikely.

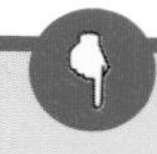

**Clinical pointers**

Diazepam is also important in preventing (and treating) seizures associated with alcohol withdrawal. The drug is often prescribed to be administered intramuscularly or rectally in order to abort seizures. Alcohol withdrawal seizures most frequently occur within 2–3 days of the commencement of withdrawal and the risk then decreases.

## Thiamine and B vitamins

Evidence suggests that the vitamin deficiencies associated with alcohol dependence require prompt treatment to prevent some of the more serious consequences.

Thiamine (vitamin $B_1$) deficiency is the most prevalent deficiency associated with alcohol dependence. Those who drink in a harmful manner should be offered thiamine supplementation. Folate and vitamin $B_{12}$ deficiencies can also be identified in the alcohol-dependent patient but the conditions are usually treated after blood tests and relevant diagnostic procedures.

### Posology, pharmacokinetics and pharmacodynamics

Thiamine is dosed orally and/or via intramuscular (IM)/intravenous (IV) injection. Products such as Pabrinex® IM/IV are used at the beginning of the detoxification process to prevent or treat Wernicke–Korsakoff Syndrome (WKS). Frequently a course of Pabrinex injections will be started alongside oral thiamine supplementation (oral supplementation alone is not guaranteed to replenish depleted thiamine to the level required). Thiamine has multiple roles in the body including the correct functioning of the nervous system, muscles and the gastro-intestinal tract. Doses of oral thiamine will typically be 100 mg three times daily. In some cases, much higher doses will be used in 'at risk' patients.

### Notable contraindications/cautions and warnings/side effects/ADRs

The Medicines and Healthcare Products Regulatory Agency (MHRA) has issued a warning with regard to injectable products such as Pabrinex because some allergic responses to its use have been noted in practice.

### Practice notes

While the CIWA-Ar scale is universally recognised, its interpretation and implementation vary between healthcare settings. Please refer to your local guidelines if asked to manage alcohol withdrawal.

Other detoxification regimes exist to manage alcohol withdrawal in dependent patients. These include what are termed 'front loading' and 'fixed dosing regimes'. Some detoxification regimes may use lorazepam or chlordiazepoxide instead of diazepam.

If patients are susceptible to seizures or have polysubstance misuse issues, anti-epileptic drugs such as carbamazepine or oxcarbazepine are often prescribed alongside the drugs discussed here.

# 29 Alcohol: maintaining abstinence

**Figure 29.1** Three entries from an in-patient medication chart illustrating how three different medications may be prescribed to assist with maintenance of abstinence from alcohol and some key features to be considered when they are administered

| REGULAR MEDICATION | | | | | Dose | |
|---|---|---|---|---|---|---|
| A | 1st date prescribed<br>12/5/2015 | Drug and form<br>Acamprosate tablets | Route | Pharmacy | 666 mg | breakfast |
| | | | | | 666 mg | lunch |
| | Prescriber's signature<br>Dr. Wiley | Other directions | | | 666 mg | high tea |
| | | | | | | night |

This drug is prescribed according to the patient's weight.

Disulfiram is one of three medications commonly used to assist patients in maintaining abstinence from the consumption of alcohol.

| REGULAR MEDICATION | | | | | Dose | |
|---|---|---|---|---|---|---|
| A | 1st date prescribed<br>12/5/2015 | Drug and form<br>Disulfiram tablets | Route<br>Oral | Pharmacy | | breakfast |
| | | | | | | lunch |
| | Prescriber's signature<br>Dr. Wiley | Other directions<br>Consume no alcohol | | | | high tea |
| | | | | | 200 mg | night |

The consumption of alcohol is contra-indicated with this medication. Drinking alcohol can lead to serious adverse effects.

Naltrexone is an opiate antagonist and influences the reward pathways in the brain. The drug will block the effect of opiates.

| REGULAR MEDICATION | | | | | Dose | |
|---|---|---|---|---|---|---|
| A | 1st date prescribed<br>12/5/2015 | Drug and form<br>Naltrexone tablets | Route<br>Oral | Pharmacy | | breakfast |
| | | | | | | lunch |
| | Prescriber's signature<br>Dr. Wiley | Other directions | | | 25 mg | high tea |
| | | | | | | night |

After undertaking a process of alcohol detoxification (Chapter 28), patients are offered options to support them in maintaining abstinence (or minimising their drinking) (Figure 29.1). Some patients spend time in a rehabilitative setting and/or are offered other packages of support. These include various psychosocial interventions and the use of medication.

Three medications are used to assist a patient in maintaining abstinence: acamprosate, disulfiram and naltrexone. There is an evidence base that supports the interventions and the medications are used either alone or in combination, depending on the wishes of the patient, their other support mechanisms and their body's ability to deal with the medication.

# Acamprosate

## Pharmacokinetics and pharmacodynamics

Acamprosate is an oral medication dosed three times daily. The dose used is dependent on the weight of the patient. Acamprosate is usually initiated after alcohol withdrawal has been undertaken and the patient is essentially abstinent. The recommended treatment period is 1 year and therapy can be continued even if relapse occurs.

Food can influence the absorption of the drug. The drug undergoes no significant hepatic metabolism and is renally excreted. The patient's renal function is one of the important influences on the suitability of using acamprosate.

The drug appears to stimulate gamma amino butyric acid (GABA) neurones and antagonises the effects of excitatory amino acids such as glutamate. This results in a decrease in the voluntary intake of alcoholic drinks.

## Notable contra-indications/cautions and warnings

The suitability of using acamprosate in those under 18 or over 65 years of age has not been tested. More severe hepatic damage, breastfeeding and renal insufficiency are important contra-indications.

## Side effects/adverse drug reactions (ADRs)

The most common side effects tend to be gastro-intestinal (GI) upset such as diarrhoea, abdominal pain and nausea. Some effects on libido are also noted in the summary of product characteristics (SPC).

# Disulfiram

## Pharmacokinetics and pharmacodynamics

Disulfiram is an oral medication that is only initiated under specialist supervision. The drug is sometimes given as a 'loading dose' but is started **after** detoxification at 200 mg per day. It must not under any circumstances be taken with alcohol. Family and/or carer support needs to be high when a patient is using disulfiram.

The drug irreversibly binds and inhibits the enzyme acetaldehyde dehydrogenase, which neutralises a toxic metabolite of alcohol. If the patient consumes alcohol while taking disufiram, this toxic metabolite accumulates within the body. This in turn leads to flushing, increased body temperature, nausea, vomiting, sweats, itchiness, palpitations and many other symptoms that are uncomfortable and unpleasant for the patient. The threat and any previous experience of this reaction is a deterrent to alcohol consumption. **Please note that this reaction can be fatal**.

## Notable contra-indications/cautions and warnings/side effects/ADRs

Consumption of alcohol is contra-indicated. There are contra-indications for cardiac conditions such as heart failure, coronary artery disease, previous cerebrovascular accidents and hypertension. Psychiatric conditions such as severe personality disorders, suicidal risk or psychosis are also contra-indicated.

Evidence of hepatic, renal, cardiac or respiratory disease is regarded as a caution for use. Cerebral damage, hypothyroidism and epilepsy are also cautions. The drug stays in the body for up to 14 days post-discontinuation and caution is required if the patient drinks alcohol during this period.

Side effects include depression, drowsiness, nausea and vomiting, fatigue and halitosis.

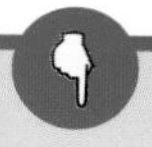

### Clinical pointers

The disulfiram–alcohol reaction may occur with other products containing alcohol, such as deodorants, mouthwashes, liquid medicines and inhalers. Care must be taken when looking after patients who may react in an adverse way to other applied products containing alcohol.

# Naltrexone

## Pharmacokinetics and pharmacodynamics

Naltrexone is an oral medication and is typically dosed at 50 mg daily. The duration of treatment is initially for 3 months but may be longer. The drug is metabolised hepatically into its active metabolite. The active metabolite and any untransformed naltrexone are both excreted renally.

Naltrexone is an opioid antagonist. The antagonism of opioid receptors in the central nervous system is believed to decrease the rewarding feeling that is associated with drinking alcohol. The drug is also used to maintain abstinence in formerly opiate-dependent patients.

## Notable contra-indications/cautions and warnings

Contra-indications to naltrexone include severe renal and hepatic impairment. Patients also using opioids cannot use naltrexone.

## Side effects/ADRs

Naltrexone can cause nausea and vomiting, GI upset and abdominal pain. The drug is associated with sleep disruption (insomnia), restlessness and agitation, mood swings and anxiety. Other common side effects include changes in liver function tests, headaches, appetite changes and increased lacrimation.

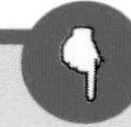

### Clinical pointers

Naltrexone can be dosed three times weekly (100 mg on Monday, 100 mg on Wednesday and 150 mg on Friday) rather than once daily. This may be helpful for patients with compliance issues such as poor social support, poor memory or who may live some distance from the healthcare professional responsible for their care.

## Practice notes

There is increasing concern that part of the health cost of alcohol consumption relates to those who drink in a harmful or hazardous fashion. These individuals may not be identified as alcoholics but will often drink at levels greater than those recommended. A recently introduced medication (nalmefene – Selincro®) has been evidenced to decrease heavy drinking in these individuals. The medication can be considered as unconventional from two perspectives. First, it is taken on an 'as required' basis. The patient takes the medication in anticipation of consuming alcohol; the result is a reduction in the amount of alcohol consumed in each drinking session, and thus the harm associated with excessive consumption. Second, it should only be prescribed in conjunction with a supportive 'psychosocial intervention'.

# Smoking cessation

**Figure 30.1** There are a range of nicotine replacement therapies available that use different means of delivery

Nicotine
nasal spray

?

Counselling

Nicotine skin patch

Bupropion sustained release

Nicotine inhalator

Nicotine gum

*Medicines Management for Nurses at a Glance*. First Edition. Simon Young and Ben Pitcher. © 2016 John Wiley & Sons, Ltd. Published 2016 by John Wiley & Sons, Ltd.
www.ataglanceseries.com/nursing/medicinesmanagement

The use of tobacco-based products has been part of our society for centuries. At one point it was believed that they were actually healthy or even curative. We know better now. The use of tobacco-based products (primarily smoking) have now been proven to be responsible for causing a large number of health problems including cancer and heart disease.

You might think that confronted with the overwhelming evidence of the harm that smoking can cause, everyone would give up smoking promptly and easily. The problem is that tobacco (and more specifically the active ingredient nicotine) is addictive.

The goals of smoking cessation are to encourage people to quit, maximise the chance of successful cessation and prevent future relapse.

## Pharmacodynamics

Nicotine is a stimulant; it is an agonist that binds to and activates a particular subtype of acetylcholine receptor. These are named nicotinic acetylcholine receptors for this reason. Nicotinic receptors are found throughout the body. However, nicotine has a higher affinity for the receptors in the brain. Because of this, at doses seen in smoking, we predominantly see effects in the brain that generally result in increased secretion of neurotransmitters, notably in the dopaminergic reward pathway. However, if the dose was high enough, activation of the nicotinic receptors in the neuromuscular junction could cause spasm and eventually respiratory paralysis.

Nicotine causes an increase in the release of excitatory neurotransmitters. If someone has been exposed to nicotine regularly for an extended period of time, their brain will have adapted to this increased level of excitation. Therefore, if the nicotine is removed, the effect of the nicotine will be missed and the level of excitation will drop below normal levels. This is what causes the symptoms of withdrawal and will remain until the brain adapts to the reduced level of excitation.

The nature of nicotine addiction is in part pharmacological, but there are also habitual processes involved with the physical act of smoking. Strategies for quitting smoking often consider both these aspects in order to maximise effectiveness (Figure 30.1).

### Potential harm

Nicotine is not harmless. It causes excitation in a variety of systems throughout the body, thereby increasing heart rate and blood pressure. It has also been shown to actively damage the vascular endothelium and it has been linked with cancer cell proliferation. However, compared with the potential damage caused by smoking, the harm it causes is negligible.

## Pharmacokinetics

### Nicotine gum/pastilles/lozenges

Delivery of nicotine via the oral route provides a relatively quick means of delivering nicotine into the blood. This approximates the 'hit' of nicotine that the patient receives when smoking, and the chewing of the gum or sucking of the sweet can help with the oral fixation aspect of smoking.

### Nicotine patches

Nicotine patches are small transdermal patches that contain a reservoir of drug that seeps out of the patch and through the skin of the patient over a period of time. They are discreet, able to be placed in an out-of-site location and, once applied, require no observable action on the part of the patient. The nature of transdermal administration means that the nicotine is delivered in a consistent fashion over a long period. The levels of nicotine in the blood are therefore consistent, preventing the peaks and troughs that can heighten the sensation of cravings.

### Nasal spray

Although not widely used, nicotine can also be administered via a nasal spray whereby it is absorbed through the mucous membranes. This allows for a rapid delivery of nicotine, which is effective in providing quick relief from cravings.

### Inhalators

Inhalators allow a patient to consume the nicotine in the same way as they would when smoking, by inhaling it. The inhalator simulates the physical act of smoking and thus satisfies the physical habit of smoking, but each 'puff' contains less nicotine than a 'puff' from a cigarette, facilitating reduction in use and avoiding the inhalation of harmful smoke products.

### Vaporators/e-cigarettes

E-cigarettes or vaporators have recently become a popular alternative strategy for smoking cessation. These devices contain a cartridge of nicotine solution that is heated and vaporised by an electric coil. This vapour (which can look like smoke) is then inhaled. Different strengths and flavours of nicotine are available, which allow the user to reduce their nicotine consumption over time.

While e-cigarettes have proved popular, there is currently limited evidence to support their effectiveness as a smoking cessation aid. They are not licensed medications and as a consequence there is limited data on their pharmacokinetics or the risk of any long-term effects. Because they are not licensed, their manufacture is not controlled in the same way as a medicine. This can result in a large variance in strength, quality and presence of additional ingredients (excipients).

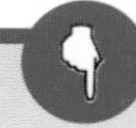

**Clinical pointers**

***Interactions***

Tobacco smoke can contain a number of chemicals that can affect the liver's capacity to metabolise certain drugs. This might result in a patient requiring higher doses of a given drug to produce the desired clinical effect. Because nicotine on its own does not have this effect, if a patient quits smoking or switches to a nicotine replacement therapy, the dose of certain drugs may need to be adjusted.

Examples include clozapine, olanzapine and theophylline.

Other drugs can be used in nicotine dependence (for example, varenciline and bupropion).

# Fighting infection

**Figure 31.1** The human body can be infected with a vast variety of organisms, from microscopic viruses and bacteria to the parasitic worms and insects that are visible to the naked eye

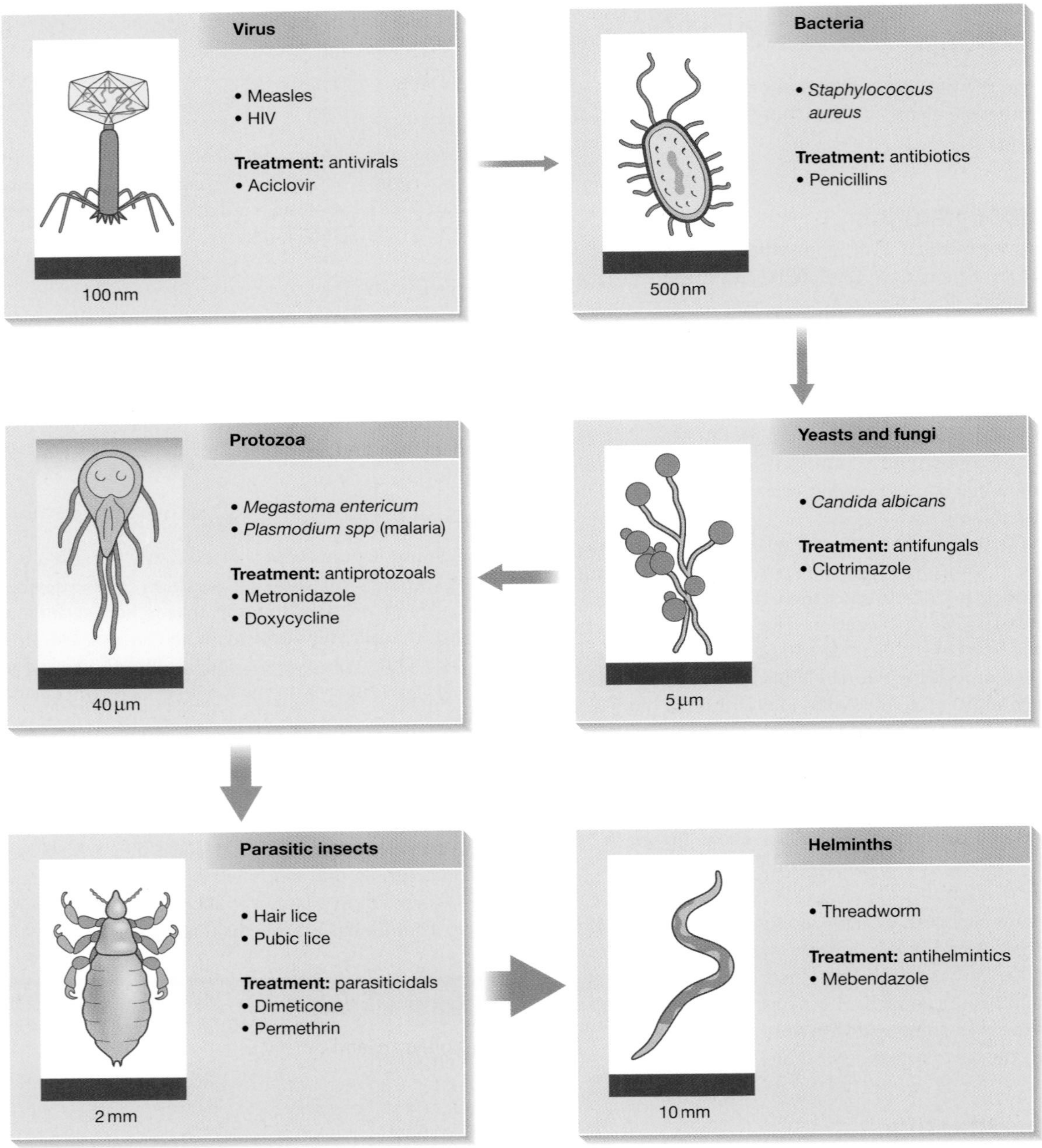

**Virus**

- Measles
- HIV

**Treatment:** antivirals
- Aciclovir

100 nm

**Bacteria**

- *Staphylococcus aureus*

**Treatment:** antibiotics
- Penicillins

500 nm

**Yeasts and fungi**

- *Candida albicans*

**Treatment:** antifungals
- Clotrimazole

5 µm

**Protozoa**

- *Megastoma entericum*
- *Plasmodium spp* (malaria)

**Treatment:** antiprotozoals
- Metronidazole
- Doxycycline

40 µm

**Parasitic insects**

- Hair lice
- Pubic lice

**Treatment:** parasiticidals
- Dimeticone
- Permethrin

2 mm

**Helminths**

- Threadworm

**Treatment:** antihelmintics
- Mebendazole

10 mm

The world is full of life, and much of it is invisible. Microscopic life forms inhabit the world around us and within us (Figure 31.1). Many of these microbes have little effect on us; some (including the large colonies of bacteria found in our bowel) are actually beneficial. However, some microbes or germs colonise and reproduce within the tissues of the body, either actively destroying cells or producing toxins that disrupt the proper functioning of our bodies.

While the threat of pathogenic organisms is everywhere, we are not defenceless. Our immune system is capable of fighting off many of the biological threats we face every day. But it has limits: there are still many circumstances in which our immune system can be overwhelmed by a pathogen. Without external help the infection could be at best unpleasant, at worst fatal.

We have therefore developed drugs to help fight infection. This has proved challenging. While it is easy to find ways to kill germs, it is hard to find ways that do not damage and kill a patient at the same time. The solution is to try and exploit the differences between microbes' cells and human cells, thereby creating a 'magic bullet' that will kill the microbes but leave the host cells untouched.

## Bacteria

**Bacteria** are single-celled prokaryotic organisms that make up most of all life on earth. They are microscopic and as a result their involvement in our world (and even their existence) was not acknowledged for most of human history.

**Antibacterials** are any agents that kill bacteria. **Antibiotics** are chemicals derived from mould that kill bacteria (although the term is often used to describe any drug that kills bacteria, regardless of its origin). It was observed that if bacteria and mould are cultured together on agar, an exclusion zone forms around the mould where the bacteria does not grow. This is because the mould produces chemicals to kill bacteria and keep its own micro-environment bacteria free. Alexander Fleming first identified this in 1929 and soon after the active chemicals involved were isolated for use in patients. Penicillin was first used clinically in the 1940s. Later research yielded additional varieties of antibiotics that work via a variety of mechanisms. Bacteria come in many sizes and shapes (morphology) that provide a means of classifying them. The morphology of bacteria provides insight into the aetiology of the diseases they may cause and which antibiotics may be most effective in treating them (see Chapter 32 for more detail).

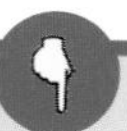

### Clinical pointers

Because antibiotics work by interfering with processes exclusively found within bacteria, they will have little or no effect on other types of organisms. This is important from two perspectives. First, antibiotics generally cause little or no harm to a patient's cells (although some toxicity is seen). Second, antibiotics will not treat fungal or viral infections (such as colds or flu).

One of the problems in modern health care is the issue of bacterial resistance. Bacteria continually evolve, developing resistance to drugs, presenting a real threat to our ability to treat infections. Antibiotics should therefore be prescribed sparingly and appropriately to slow the development of resistance.

## Viruses

**Viruses** are significantly smaller than bacteria. They are small packets of genetic material that reproduce by entering cells and hijack the cellular machinery, using it to produce more viruses. This continues until there are so many viruses in the cell that it ruptures and releases them.

**Antiviral** drugs are often used to treat severe or persistent viral infections such as HIV, cytomegalovirus, and also topically to treat herpes simplex (cold sores). In general, antivirals are used less often than antibiotics because simple viral infections (such as colds) will be fought off by the immune system and immunisation schedules have reduced the impact and burden of more severe viral illnesses (e.g. measles).

There are comparatively few antiviral drugs available and most act by inhibiting the enzymes used by the viruses to insert their genetic material into our cellular machinery. Inhibiting these enzymes prevents a virus from reproducing.

## Fungi

**Fungi** are a large family of organisms that include mushrooms and toadstools. However, there are also a large number of microscopic fungi, such as yeasts and moulds. It is possible for these to infect the body.

**Antifungal** agents exploit the differences between fungal cells and our own. However, fungal cells are less different from our own (compared with bacteria), which presents additional challenges in finding ways to kill a fungus without harming the patient. Types of fungal infection include athlete's foot, thrush and ringworm.

## Other organisms

**Protozoa** are single-celled eukaryotic organisms that are found in fluid or moist environments. They are often associated with disease and are the cause of malaria. **Antiprotozoal drugs** are not used very commonly in the UK. However, globally they are used extensively, especially in tropical regions where malaria is endemic.

There are a variety of more complex organisms that can infest the human body. **Parasitic worms** are not microscopic, but their eggs often are and can enter the body through our food, growing as they feed off us. **Antihelmintics** are drugs used to deal with infestations of worms and other parasitic organisms.

Examples of other infestations include head lice and scabies.

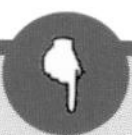

### Clinical pointer

Because we are not always aware of which patient might be infected or infested, we must always ensure that we consider universal precautions for the prevention of cross-infection.

# 32 Antibiotics

**Figure 32.1** Two entries from an in-patient medication chart illustrating how co-amoxiclav and gentamicin may be prescribed and some key features to be considered when they are administered

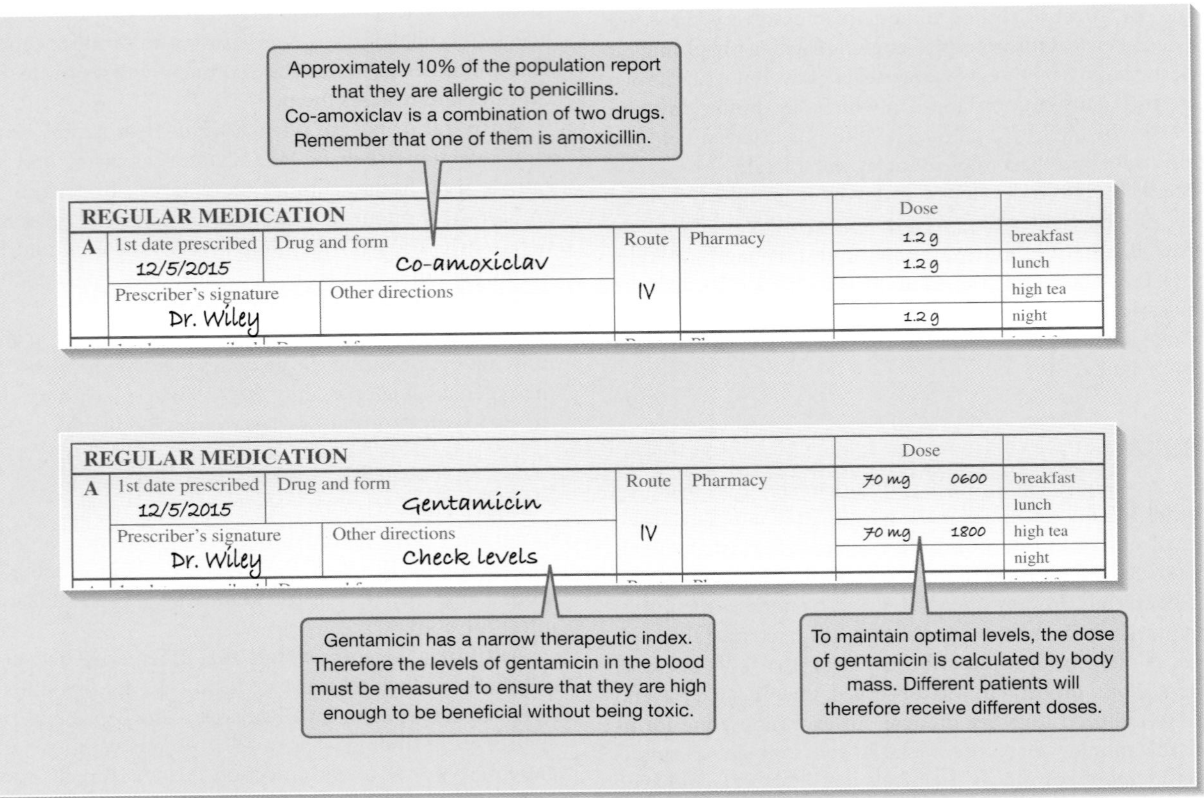


**Figure 32.2** Diagram of β-lactam ring structure common to some antibiotics

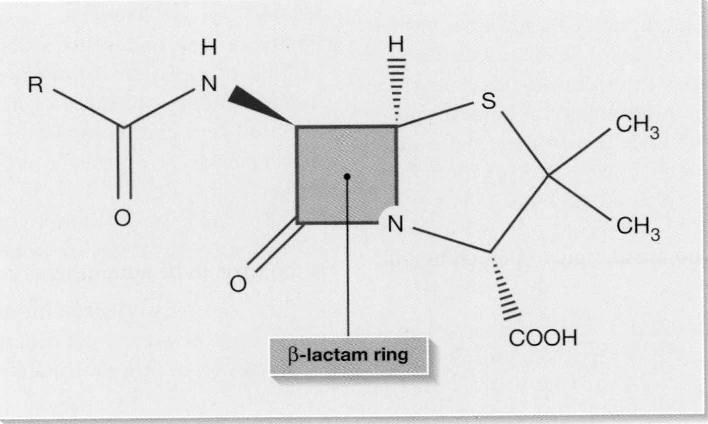


As discussed in Chapter 31, antibiotics are important tools for helping us survive bacterial infections, supporting our own immune system that might otherwise be overwhelmed. There are several families or groups of antibiotics that are used (Figure 32.1). Each group has a different mechanism of action and is effective against different strains of bacteria. Those antibiotics that are effective against a wide range of bacteria are called 'broad-spectrum' antibiotics and are used when the exact nature of the infection is not known.

*Medicines Management for Nurses at a Glance*. First Edition. Simon Young and Ben Pitcher.  Published 2016 by John Wiley & Sons, Ltd.
www.ataglanceseries.com/nursing/medicinesmanagement

## Penicillins

### Common examples

- Benzylpenicillin.
- Flucloxacillin.
- Amoxicillin.
- Ampicillin.

### Indications

Penicillins are some of the oldest and most widely used antibiotics available. They are indicated the treatment or prophylaxis of a wide variety of bacterial threats.

### Pharmacodynamics

As discussed in the previous chapter, antibiotics work by exploiting the differences between bacterial cells and the cells of our body. One particular difference is that most bacteria have a peptidoglycan cell wall. Penicillins interfere with the synthesis of the cell wall, which prevents the bacteria from growing properly, resulting in their death.

A key feature common to the molecular structure of penicillins is the beta-lactam ring (Figure 32.2). It is this structure that inhibits the synthesis of the peptidoglycan wall.

### Pharmacokinetics

Penicillins are administered by oral or injectable routes.

### Side effects/adverse drug reactions (ADRs)

The most notable adverse drug reaction associated with penicillins is allergy. Research indicates that between 1 in 10 and 1 in 100 patients experience some form of allergy (usually skin rash). The more serious and potentially life-threatening anaphylaxis is far less common (approximately 1 in 2000). It is important to remember that patients who have demonstrated allergy to one form of penicillin are highly likely to be allergic to all members of this group. Patients who have exhibited a severe and immediate reaction to penicillin may also have allergy to other types of antibiotic that share the beta-lactam ring structure.

## Cephalosporins

### Common examples

- Cefuroxime.
- Cefotaxime.
- Ceftriaxone.
- Ceftazidime.

Cephalosporins are widely used for the treatment and prophylaxis of a variety of bacterial threats. While chemically distinct from penicillin, they also contain a beta-lactam ring that allows them to prevent bacterial synthesis of the peptidoglycan wall. Like penicillin, some patients can be allergic to cephalosporins. Approximately 5% of patients who are allergic to penicillin will also be allergic to cephalosporins.

## Other beta-lactam antibiotics

There are a variety of other beta-lactam antibiotics that are less commonly used. These include the carbapenems – for example, meropenem and imipenem.

## Beta-lactamases and inhibitors

Bacteria have the capacity to mutate. Useful mutations allow bacteria to prosper and the mutation becomes the new norm. Bacterial mutations can result in resistance to antibiotics. One such example of this type of mutation is the evolution of beta-lactmases. These enzymes bind to and inhibit the action of the beta-lactam ring, neutralising the effect of the antibiotic. To combat this, we have developed beta-lactamase inhibitors that prevent the action of the beta-lactamase enzymes and allow the antibiotic to be effective. Beta-lactamase inhibitors are often combined with antibiotics in a single formulation such as co-amoxiclav, which combines the antibiotic amoxicillin with the beta-lactamase inhibitor clavulinic acid.

## Tetracyclines

### Common example

- Doxycycline.

Antibiotics target differences between bacterial cells and our own cells. This allows them to be toxic to the bacteria but less toxic to us. The bacterial ribosome is different from ours and as such is a useful pharmacological target. Tetracyclines inhibit the binding of the 30S subunit of the bacterial ribosome, thereby preventing the expression of genes and the synthesising of bacterial proteins. Tetracyclines can be used for a variety of infections, but are often seen in treating genito-urinary infections and acne. Tetracyclines should not be given to pregnant or breastfeeding mothers or to young children because they affect the formation of bones and teeth.

## Macrolides

### Common examples

- Erythromycin.
- Clarithromycin.
- Azithromycin.

Macrolides attach to the 50S subunit of the bacterial ribosome. They are broad-spectrum antibiotics and useful as an alternative to penicillin in patients who are either allergic to penicillin or whose infection is penicillin resistant. Macrolides (erythromycin especially) commonly cause abdominal discomfort, diarrhoea and gastro-intestinal (GI) distress. These antibiotics can be administered orally, intravenously or topically for acne. When administered intravenously, they can be caustic (particularly clarithromycin) and cause irritation at the infusion site.

## Aminoglycosides

### Common examples:

- Gentamicin.
- Neomycin.

Aminoglycosides interfere with protein synthesis within the bacterial cell. They are powerful and fast acting, and used to treat serious infections of an unknown nature. They are also quite toxic causing damage to the kidneys and the inner ear. Serum gentamicin levels must be monitored to keep toxicity to a minimum. Neomycin is too toxic to be administered parenterally: it is most commonly applied directly to infected skin or mucous membranes.

## Metronidazole

Metronidazole is a broad-spectrum antibiotic effective against anaerobic bacterial infections. It is commonly used as a prophylactic to protect surgical patients from infection. It is often stated that you should not consume alcohol while on antibiotics but most of the time it does little harm. However, patients taking metronidazole should never consume alcohol. Metronidazole inhibits an enzyme that is used in the metabolism of alcohol, resulting in a build-up of acetaldehyde that can cause a variety of unpleasant side effects including vasodilation, tachycardia, dyspnoea, electrocardiogram (ECG) changes, nausea, vomiting, headache, convulsions and coma. These effects are similar to those of the drug disulfiram (Chapter 29).

# 33 Diabetes: insulin

**Figure 33.1** A graph illustrating endogenous insulin production over the course of a typical day. The peaks correspond to the increases in insulin produced in response to eating a meal

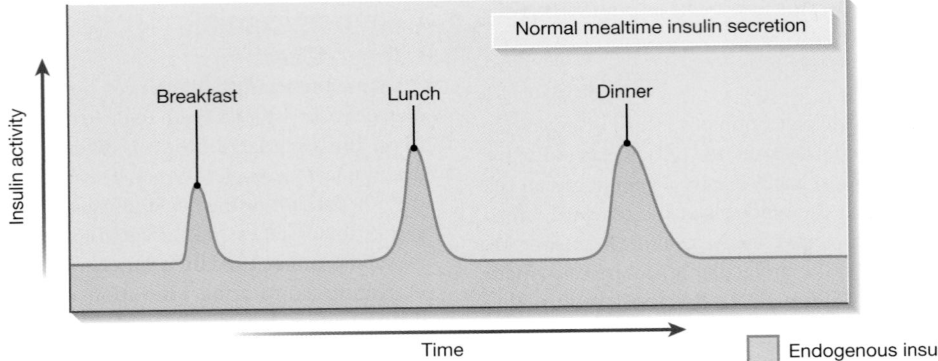


**Figure 33.2** A graph illustrating how a basal-bolus regime of insulin dosing attempts to mimic the pattern of insulin production seen in a healthy individual

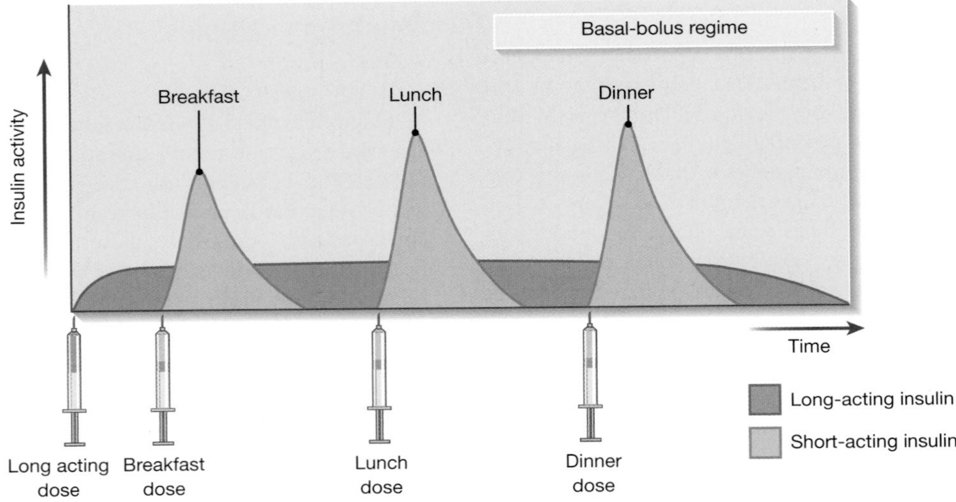


**Figure 33.3** A graph illustrating how a twice-daily pre-mixed regime of insulin dosing attempts to mimic the pattern of insulin production seen in a healthy individual

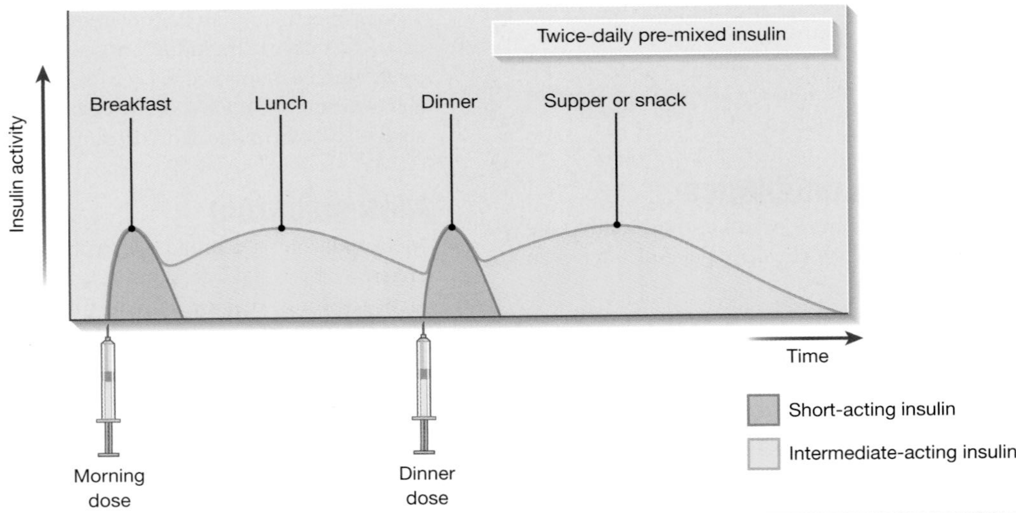

Diabetes mellitus is a disease that is defined by a reduced ability to produce insulin, or an insensitivity of the cells of the body to the insulin that is produced. This results in an inability to use or store glucose absorbed from the digestive system. If diabetes mellitus is not properly treated, it can have potentially debilitating and life-shortening outcomes.

Diabetes can be categorised into different types according to its presentation and cause. Certain types of diabetes tend to be treated by certain types of drugs. This resulted in diabetes being classified by how it was treated (insulin dependent or non-insulin dependent). However, this system is no longer used because it is an over-simplification of the complexities of the disease and its varied treatment strategies.

The main types of diabetes:

Type 1

- Complete loss of insulin production from the beta cells of the islets of Langerhans.
- Tends to manifest early in life.
- Predominantly treated with insulin and controlled diet.

Type 2

- Reduced production of insulin or reduced sensitivity of the body's tissues to the insulin that is produced.
- Accounts for approximately 90% of all diabetes.
- Tends to manifest later in life (although can occur in children).
- Can be treated with diet and exercise, oral antidiabetic medication or insulin.

Gestational diabetes

- Inability of a pregnant woman's body to produce enough insulin to account for the reduced insulin sensitivity of the tissues caused by various pregnancy hormones.
- Raises additional problems because of the need to treat diabetes without harming the foetus.

# Insulins

## Indications

At the heart of diabetes is an insufficient supply of insulin. If the body is not producing enough insulin (or none at all), the most straightforward solution is to supply the missing insulin from an external source.

## Pharmacodynamics

Insulin is a protein (comprised of 51 amino acids) produced by the islets of Langerhans in the pancreas. It plays an important role in regulating the level of glucose within the blood. In healthy individuals blood sugars rise after eating food. Insulin is then released from the pancreas to allow the glucose to be used by the cells of the body and to be taken up into the liver to be stored as glycogen.

The earliest forms of insulin therapy were extracted from animals such as cows (bovine insulin) and pigs (porcine insulin). These are almost identical to human insulin, differing by only three and one amino acids respectively. Animal insulins have been associated with allergy and patients developing resistance to their effects. More recently, we have been able to genetically modify bacteria to synthesise exact copies of human insulin or to produce insulin with specific beneficial differences.

These differences to the structure of insulin, or what it is bound to, can affect the rate at which the insulin is absorbed, and therefore how long a single administration continues to have effect. These can be grouped into three categories: short acting (e.g. Actrapid®), intermediate acting (e.g. isophane insulin) and long acting (e.g. insulin glargine).

## Pharmacokinetics

Insulin is a protein and as such cannot be taken orally. If it is swallowed, the acids and enzymes of the digestive tract would destroy it. As a result it must be administered via a parenteral route. For most patients this is done via subcutaneous injection (or occasionally infusion); however, seriously ill patients may be administered insulin intravenously.

Dosing of insulin must be undertaken **very** carefully: if too little is given, the patient may develop hyperglycaemia. If too much is given, the patient may become hypoglycaemic. In health, insulin is released from the pancreas in response to rising glucose in the blood. The amount released is continually titrated as part of a negative feedback system designed to keep the blood sugar within tightly controlled limits. The pancreas typically releases a baseline level of insulin throughout the day. As blood sugars increase in response to eating food, insulin production is increased (Figure 33.1).

Mimicking this tight control with externally administered insulin is very difficult. Careful selection and combination of different types of insulin can produce a number of regimes for managing diabetes.

### Basal-bolus regime

This regime incorporates a single injection of a long-acting insulin (e.g. Lantus®), which provides a baseline (or basal) level of insulin. Additional injections (or boluses) of short-acting insulin are then administered at each meal to account for the increase in blood sugar (Figure 33.2). While this system allows a lot of control, it requires multiple injections of different types of insulin, which may be confusing.

### Twice-daily pre-mixed biphasic

This system uses pre-mixed insulin preparations that combine short-acting and intermediate-acting insulin in a single solution. This means that a single injection will produce two peaks of insulin in the patient – one immediately after administration and one a few hours later. The patient is given insulin for the whole day (including covering four meals) with only two injections (Figure 33.3). However, this regime can cause challenges for individuals with less predictable lives.

### Continuous infusion

The continuous infusion of insulin allows the use of short-acting insulin to be given at a rate that will keep the blood sugars within a target range. A patient's blood sugars are checked regularly and the rate of infusion adjusted, using what is referred to as a sliding scale. Historically, continuous infusion of insulin was only done in hospital with acutely unwell patients. However, in recent years, small battery-powered insulin pumps have been used to supply short-acting insulin continuously through the day for patients in the community.

## Side effects/adverse drug reactions (ADRs)

Beyond the obvious potential for overdose, insulin can cause hypokaelemia as well as lipodystrophy (unsightly wasting of the fatty tissue at the site of injection).

# Diabetes: antiglycaemics

**Figure 34.1** An entry from an in-patient medication chart illustrating how antiglycaemics may be prescribed and some key features to be considered when it is administered

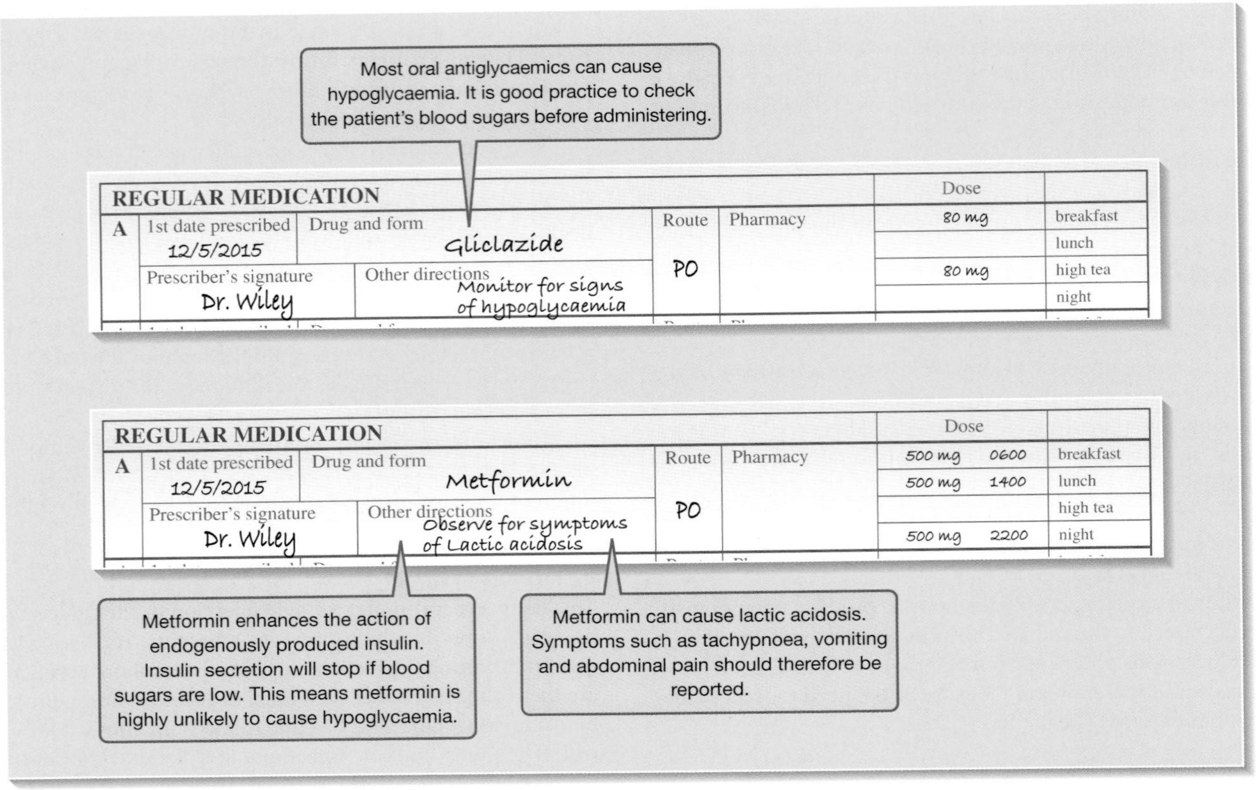

Most oral antiglycaemics can cause hypoglycaemia. It is good practice to check the patient's blood sugars before administering.

| REGULAR MEDICATION | | | | | Dose | |
|---|---|---|---|---|---|---|
| A | 1st date prescribed 12/5/2015 | Drug and form Gliclazide | Route PO | Pharmacy | 80 mg | breakfast |
| | | | | | | lunch |
| | Prescriber's signature Dr. Wiley | Other directions Monitor for signs of hypoglycaemia | | | 80 mg | high tea |
| | | | | | | night |

| REGULAR MEDICATION | | | | | Dose | |
|---|---|---|---|---|---|---|
| A | 1st date prescribed 12/5/2015 | Drug and form Metformin | Route PO | Pharmacy | 500 mg 0600 | breakfast |
| | | | | | 500 mg 1400 | lunch |
| | Prescriber's signature Dr. Wiley | Other directions Observe for symptoms of Lactic acidosis | | | | high tea |
| | | | | | 500 mg 2200 | night |

Metformin enhances the action of endogenously produced insulin. Insulin secretion will stop if blood sugars are low. This means metformin is highly unlikely to cause hypoglycaemia.

Metformin can cause lactic acidosis. Symptoms such as tachypnoea, vomiting and abdominal pain should therefore be reported.

Diabetes is the inability of the body to produce adequate amounts of insulin, resulting in an inability to correctly use glucose. The most obvious way to treat this condition is to administer insulin (or insulin analogues) to replace what would normally be produced by the pancreas (Chapter 33). However, in type 2 diabetes, the pancreas retains some function and is able to produce some insulin. For patients with type 2 diabetes, there are a variety of drug therapies that can be used to increase insulin secretion, increase the insulin's effectiveness or reduce blood sugar by preventing its absorption or expediting its clearance from the body (Figure 34.1).

The British National Formulary (BNF) classifies these drugs into the following groups:

- Biguanides.
- Sulfonylureas.
- 'Other' antidiabetics.

## Biguanides

The only available member of this group is metformin.

### Indications

Metformin is used alone or in combination with other therapies for the treatment of type 2 diabetes.

### Pharmacodynamics

Metformin activates an important liver enzyme called AMP-activated protein kinase (AMPK).

AMPK has a wide range of effects, including increasing insulin sensitivity, increasing use of glucose, decreasing absorption of glucose from the intestine and inhibiting the synthesis of glucose from smaller biochemicals (gluconeogenesis). Metformin will only trigger these effects in the presence of insulin. This means that a patient must have at least a partially functioning pancreas that is able to produce some insulin. It also means that metformin is highly unlikely to cause hypoglycaemia. If the blood sugar levels drop too low, the pancreas will stop producing insulin and the drug will cease its effect.

### Pharmacokinetics

As with most antidiabetic drugs, metformin is taken orally.

### Side effects/adverse drug reactions (ADRs)

Metformin is also known to produce a variety of gastro-intestinal (GI) side effects, including nausea, vomiting and abdominal pain.

### Notable contra-indications/cautions and warnings

Metformin may provoke **lactic acidosis**, especially in patients who have renal impairment. Lactic acidosis is the build-up of lactic acid in the body. The signs of lactic acidosis are drowsiness, deep and rapid breathing, vomiting and abdominal pain.

### Clinical pointer

Metformin is usually given with food to minimise gastro intestinal side effects.

## Sulfonylureas

- Glibenclamide.
- Gliclazide.

### Indications

These are used in type 2 diabetes, particularly in patients who have not tolerated metformin. Several agents are available and choice depends on factors such as age, renal function and side effects.

### Pharmacodynamics

Sulfonylureas bind to potassium channels on the membrane of beta cells in the islets of Langerhans. By facilitating an efflux of potassium and a subsequent influx of calcium, they trigger the release of insulin from the cell. This means that sulfonylureas need functioning beta cells to have an effect.

### Pharmacokinetics

As with most antidiabetic drugs, sulfonylureas are taken orally.

### Side effects/ADRs

Sulfonylureas trigger insulin release regardless of the current blood sugar levels. As a result, unlike metformin, they can cause hypoglycaemia. This typically indicates that the dose is too large.

## 'Other' antidiabetics

### Acarbose

Acarbose inhibits an enzyme that results in a delay in the digestion and absorption of starch and sucrose. This has a small but significant effect in lowering blood glucose. It can be used alone or in combination with other antidiabetic drugs (e.g. metformin). Because it prevents the absorption of sugars from the intestine, the flora of the large bowel feed upon it causing flatulence.

### Nateglinide and repaglinide

These are classed as post-prandial (after-meal) controllers. They are taken up to 30 minutes before a meal to 'control' the post-prandial blood sugar spike that occurs as a meal is digested. Poor control of these post-prandial blood sugar spikes may be linked to complications associated with diabetes. Nateglinide and repaglinide reduce these spikes by stimulating insulin release. They are usually taken with or before a meal and can be omitted if the meal is missed, thereby helping to prevent hypoglycaemia.

## Incretin mimetics

- Exenatide.
- Liraglutide.
- Lixisenatide.

Incretins are protein hormones, produced by the small intestine, which help to regulate appetite and the secretion of insulin. When food enters the duodenum, incretins are released to enhance the secretion of insulin from the pancreas. The incretins are then quickly broken down by an enzyme, dipeptidyl peptidase-4 (DPP-4). This is part of the body's mechanism for preventing post-prandial sugar spikes. Incretin mimetics were originally derived from the saliva of a Gila monster, a type of lizard. Because the lizard's incretins are subtly different from human incretins, the enzymes that break it down are less effective, allowing it to remain active for longer. It is a protein-based drug, so it cannot be taken orally or it would be destroyed by the patient's digestive enzymes; it is therefore only available as a subcutaneous injection.

## DPP-4 inhibitors

- Sitagliptin.
- Linagliptin.
- Saxagliptin.
- Vildagliptin.

As discussed earlier, incretins enhance the release of insulin from the pancreas in response to consuming food. The DPP-4 enzyme breaks down the incretins to switch off this mechanism. DPP-4 inhibitors prevent the incretins from being broken down, extending the duration of their effect and increasing the amount of insulin released by the pancreas. Unlike the incretin mimetics, the DPP-4 inhibitors are not protein based and can therefore be administered orally.

## Pioglitazone (Actos®)

This is a member of a group of drugs called the thiazolidinediones. They enhance the expression of certain genes within a cell; one of the outcomes of this is reduced peripheral insulin resistance. This facilitates a reduction in blood-glucose concentration. However, there are concerns regarding the side effects of this drug, including increased cardiovascular risk and risk of cancer.

# Thyroid conditions

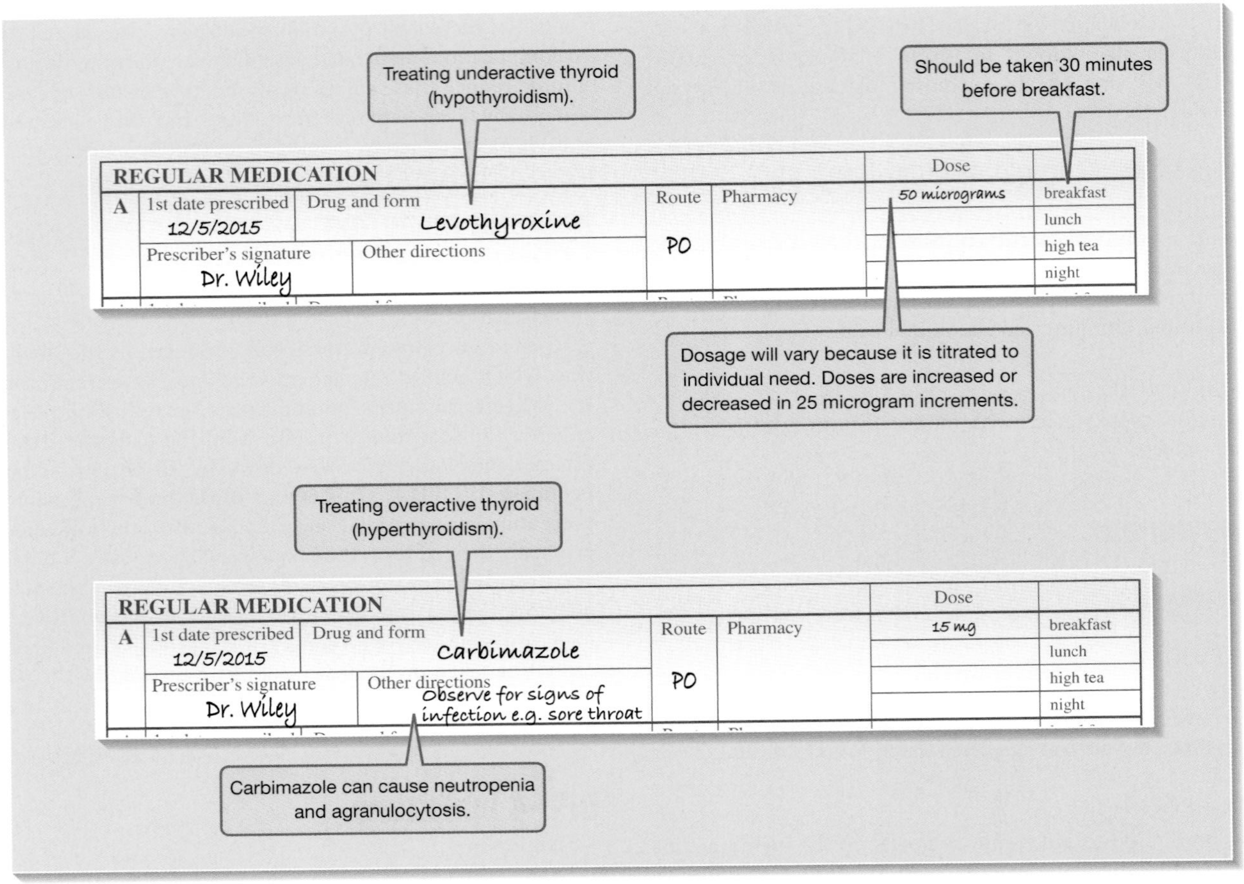

Figure 35.1 An entry from an in-patient medication chart illustrating how levothyroxine and carbimazole may be prescribed and some key features to be considered when it is administered


Treating underactive thyroid (hypothyroidism).
Should be taken 30 minutes before breakfast.
REGULAR MEDICATION
Dose
A
1st date prescribed
12/5/2015
Drug and form
Levothyroxine
Route
PO
Pharmacy
50 micrograms
breakfast
lunch
high tea
night
Prescriber's signature
Dr. Wiley
Other directions
Dosage will vary because it is titrated to individual need. Doses are increased or decreased in 25 microgram increments.
Treating overactive thyroid (hyperthyroidism).
REGULAR MEDICATION
Dose
A
1st date prescribed
12/5/2015
Drug and form
Carbimazole
Route
PO
Pharmacy
15 mg
breakfast
lunch
high tea
night
Prescriber's signature
Dr. Wiley
Other directions
Observe for signs of infection e.g. sore throat
Carbimazole can cause neutropenia and agranulocytosis.

The thyroid gland is situated in the neck, below the larynx. It produces the thyroid hormones that play an important role in regulating the body's metabolic rate.

The two main thyroid hormones are **tetraiodothyronine ($T_4$)** – often called **thyroxine** and **triiodothyronine ($T_3$)**. In normal healthy thyroid activity (euthyroid), approximately 20 times as much $T_4$ is produced as $T_3$.

$T_4$ stimulates the cardiovascular system, augmenting the influence of the sympathetic nervous system. This increases the cardiac output and respiratory rate, and raises the basal metabolic rate.

$T_3$ enhances the breakdown of proteins, lipids and glycogen. By increasing the number of beta-adrenergic receptors in the myocardium, it also causes an increase in blood pressure. It has been linked with increasing levels of serotonin (5-HT) in the brain.

The thyroid hormones help to maintain homeostasis. Their production and release need to be tightly controlled to avoid over- or under-stimulating the metabolism. Over-production of thyroid hormones is called 'hyperthyroidism' and under-secretion is called 'hypothyroidism'. Both these pathological states can occur and be managed with pharmacological interventions (Figure 35.1).

## Hypothyroidism

### Levothyroxine and levothyronine. Indications

The under-secretion of thyroid hormones is also referred to as **underactive thyroid**. This can be caused by insufficient availability of the raw material used to synthesise the hormones (such as iodine), or by damage to the gland itself. In some patients, the body's immune system attacks the tissue of the gland causing thyroiditis. Damage can also be the result of treatments for thyroid cancer or to manage hyperthyroidism.

Patients suffering with hypothyroidism will complain of fatigue, weight gain, depression, aching muscles, dry skin and brittle hair.

### Pharmacodynamics

Pharmacological interventions for hypothyroidism revolve around providing replacement thyroid hormones. Levothyroxine is a synthetic form of $T_4$ and liothyronine is a synthetic form of $T_3$. As such, the mechanism of action of these agents is identical to those of the endogenously created hormones.

### Pharmacokinetics

Levothyroxine and liothyronine are available in tablet form, although liothyronine can be administered intravenously in severe cases. Levothyronine has a faster onset of action but is also metabolised faster, which can make it harder to maintain stable serum concentrations of the drug.

### Side effects/adverse drug reactions (ADRs)

At optimal dosing levels, side effects are minimal; however, if dosing is in excess of that required, patients can develop symptoms of hyperthyroidism such as tachycardia, arrhythmia, restlessness, excitability and insomnia. Patients may also experience gastro-intestinal (GI) disturbances.

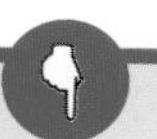

#### Clinical pointers

At present, levothyronine is not recommended for the treatment of standard hypothyroidism in preference to levothyroxine. All patients on levothyroxine (even if the condition is stable) will require at least annual blood tests to check adherence and appropriateness of dose.

## Antithyroid drugs

Hyperthyroidism can be treated in many ways. Interventions include surgery of the thyroid gland, radioactive iodine therapies and the use of antithyroid agents. The most appropriate interventions (or combination of interventions) are based on considerations such as the cause of excessive thyroid hormone production and other patient-related factors. The most commonly used antithyroid agents are carbimazole and propylthiouracil.

### Carbimazole

#### *Pharmacokinetics and pharmacodynamics*

Carbimazole is typically administered as an oral tablet. The drug is available in 5 mg and 20 mg denominations. It is usually administered as a **maintenance regimen** or a **blocking-replacement regimen**. The maintenance regimen involves an initial dose, usually in the range of 15–40 mg until the patient is euthyroid, followed by a reduction to a typically lower maintenance dose for between 6 and 18 months. The blocking-replacement regimen involves the co-administration of an initial dose of carbimazole (15–40 mg) with levothyroxine to prevent the patient becoming hypothyroid. The drug is administered (daily or as split doses) according to specific regimens. It acts by suppressing the synthesis of thyroid hormones in the body.

#### *Notable contra-indications/cautions and warnings*

The drug is contra-indicated to severe blood disorders. It can affect foetal development and passes into breast milk.

#### *Side effects*

Typical side effects include nausea, GI disturbances, taste disturbance, headache, fever, malaise, rash, pruritus and arthralgia. There is a warning in the British National Formulary (BNF) because carbimazole can cause bone marrow suppression:

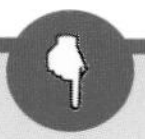

#### Clinical pointers

Warn patient to tell the doctor ***immediately*** if sore throat, mouth ulcers, bruising, fever, malaise, or non-specific illness develops.

### Propylthiouracil

#### *Pharmacokinetics and pharmacodynamics*

Propylthiouracil is an oral medication. The drug is available in 50 mg denominations. Initially it is dosed in the range 300–600 mg daily, either once daily or in divided doses until the patient becomes euthyroid. When the condition is controlled (usually after 1–2 months), the dose is reduced to 50–150 mg daily and continued for 1–2 years. The drug acts by suppressing the synthesis of thyroid hormones in the body. It may take some weeks to see its effect.

#### *Notable contra-indications/cautions and warnings*

The drug has no contra-indications except hypersensitivity; however, it is hepatotoxic and medical staff should be aware of monitoring hepatic function. Both patients and staff should be aware of the signs and symptoms of declining liver function and hepatic disorders.

#### *Side effects*

The side effects of the drug are not dissimilar to those of carbimazole, including a link to blood disorders.

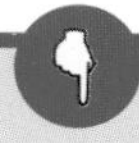

#### Clinical pointers

The beta-blocker, propranolol, is often used in severe hyperthyroidism. The beta-blocking action protects the body from the stimulating effects of the thyroxine.

# 36 Oral contraception

**Figure 36.1** An entry from an in-patient medication chart illustrating how a hormonal contraceptive (microgynon) may be prescribed, and some key features to be considered when it is administered

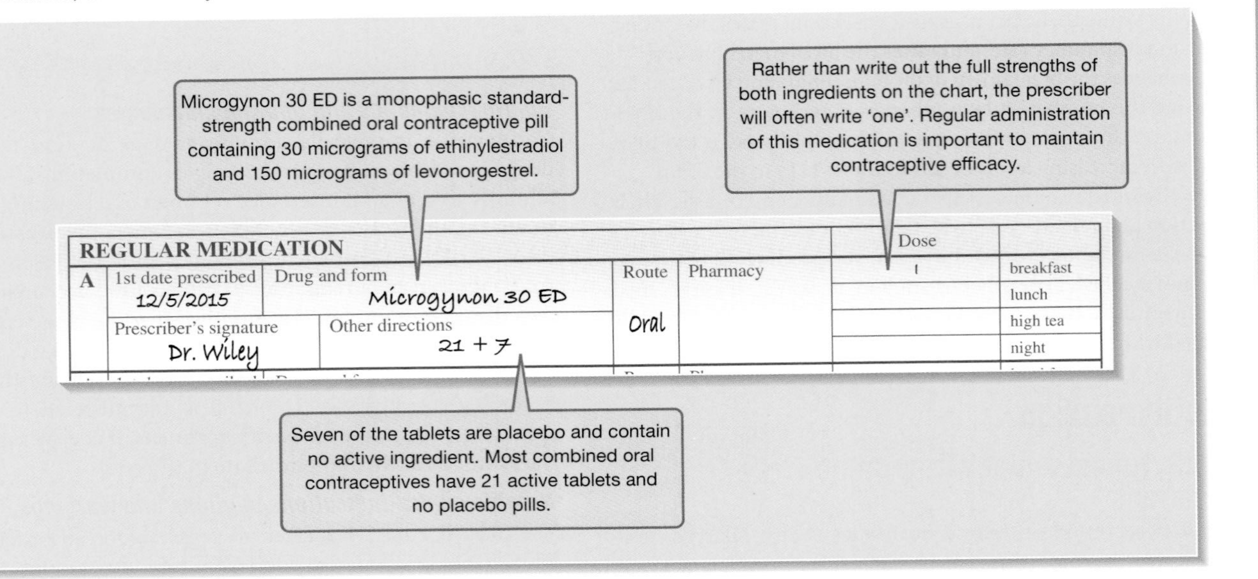

Many forms of contraception are available to patients in the UK. Contraceptives are not only used to control fertility: they are also a means of treating menstrual disorders and, in the case of barrier methods, protecting the participant from sexually transmitted infections (such as HIV). This section will focus on hormonal contraception and some of the clinical issues associated with their use (Figure 36.1).

## Hormonal contraception

Hormonal contraceptives are generally accepted to be a reliable method of birth control. As with all medication, there are a number of side effects and contra-indications that mean they are more suitable for some women than others. There are also interactions between hormonal contraceptives and other medication(s) that make them particularly challenging to manage for some women. Gastro-intestinal (GI) disturbance (e.g. vomiting, severe diarrhoea) or the use of some antibiotics can reduce the efficacy of oral contraceptive pills. The British National Formulary (BNF) monograph and summary of product characteristics (SPC) for each medication give specific details on this matter.

Hormonal contraception is available via different routes: oral tablets, parenteral preparations (depot injections and implants), transdermal patches and vaginal ring devices.

## Medications

Oral contraceptives are classified as combined hormonal or progestogen only.

**Combined hormonal contraceptives** contain two hormone types: oestrogens and progestogens.

Most combined hormonal contraceptives have ethinylestradiol as the oestrogenic component. An ethinylestradiol concentration in the range of 30–40 micrograms is used in standard-strength pills. Low-strength pills containing 20 micrograms of ethinylestradiol are more appropriate for use by women with risk factors (see later) associated with combined hormonal contraceptive use. The hormones desogestrel, gestodene and drospirenone are examples of the most frequently used progestogenic components.

The choice of pill depends on the patient and other factors such as concordance, lifestyle and other medical conditions.

### Logynon®

#### Pharmacokinetics and pharmacodynamics

Combined oral contraceptives are typically taken once daily for 21 days and no medication is taken for the next 7 days ('pill-free interval'). Hormonal contraceptives are recommended to be taken about the same time each day. If a pill is missed, contraceptive efficacy is maintained if the pill is taken within 12 hours of the correct time of administration.

The medication prevents pregnancy by:

- changing the body's hormonal balance to prevent ovulation
- thinning the lining of the womb
- thickening mucous made by the cervix, thereby forming a mucous plug.

#### Notable contra-indications/cautions and warnings

There is an extensive list of contra-indications associated with combined hormonal contraceptive use – for example, existing or history of confirmed thromoboembolism, stroke, myocardial infarction, angina, severe or multiple risk factors associated with venous thromboembolic disease, severe or uncontrolled hypertension, history of migraine with focal symptoms, severe diabetes (with vascular changes), certain hepatic diseases and current or historical breast cancer.

The BNF and SPCs clearly list a series of signs, symptoms and medical presentations that warrant the immediate stopping of oral contraception. It is important to be aware of these factors when caring for patients using combined hormonal contraception (or hormone replacement therapy). In addition, there are several risk factors that are cautions associated with combined oral contraceptive use.

#### Side effects/adverse drug reactions (ADRs)

The most common side effects include nausea, vomiting and abdominal cramping. Others include issues associated with thromboembolic disease and liver disease, mood-related issues including depression and libido changes, and others such as 'spotting' and changes in menstrual loss.

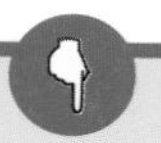

**Clinical pointers**

Some patients will use everyday (ED) pills. They will take active pills for 21 days and then 7 days of inactive/placebo pills (containing no hormone). ED pills are used primarily to assist with concordance. Please read the BNF carefully when caring for a patient using combined hormonal contraception whether it is oral, a patch or a vaginal ring.

### Progestogen-only contraceptives

Progestogen-only contraceptives (POPs) contain hormones such as desogestrel, norethisterone and levonorgestrel, and **have no oestrogenic component**.

#### Pharmacokinetics and pharmacodynamics

POPs are typically taken once daily for 28 days. As with the combined hormonal contraceptives, they are recommended to be taken about the same time each day. If a pill is missed, contraceptive efficacy is maintained if the pill is taken within a fixed time period, usually between 3 and 12 hours of the correct time of administration.

The progestogen-based contraceptives act by a combination of inhibition of ovulation and increased viscosity of the cervical mucus (dependent on the hormone present).

#### Notable contra-indications/cautions and warnings

There are comparatively fewer specific contra-indications to POP use than combined hormonal contraceptives. Those most frequently quoted are undiagnosed vaginal bleeding, severe arterial disease and a history of breast cancer.

#### Side effects/ADRs

Side effects are menstrual irregularities, nausea, vomiting, headaches and dizziness in addition to changes in mood and libido. There is a small risk association between breast cancer and the use of POPs.

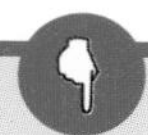

**Clinical pointers**

Parenteral POPs are used in practice. These are depot injections with contraceptive activity that lasts for longer durations, such as 8 weeks in the case of norethisterone enantate (Noristerat®). Implants such as Nexplanon® provide contraception for up to 3 years. Patients using these methods need to be counselled as to the duration of action. The side effects, contra-indications and cautions are similar to those quoted for the oral POP preparations. The method of delivery may have its own local effects. Progestogen-only intra-uterine devices are also used in practice for the treatment of menstrual disorders and contraceptive purposes.

# 37 Anticoagulants

Figure 37.1 A diagram illustrating how warfarin acts on vitamin K epoxide reductase, preventing the activation of vitamin K that is needed by the vitamin K-dependent carboxylase to activate crucial clotting factors

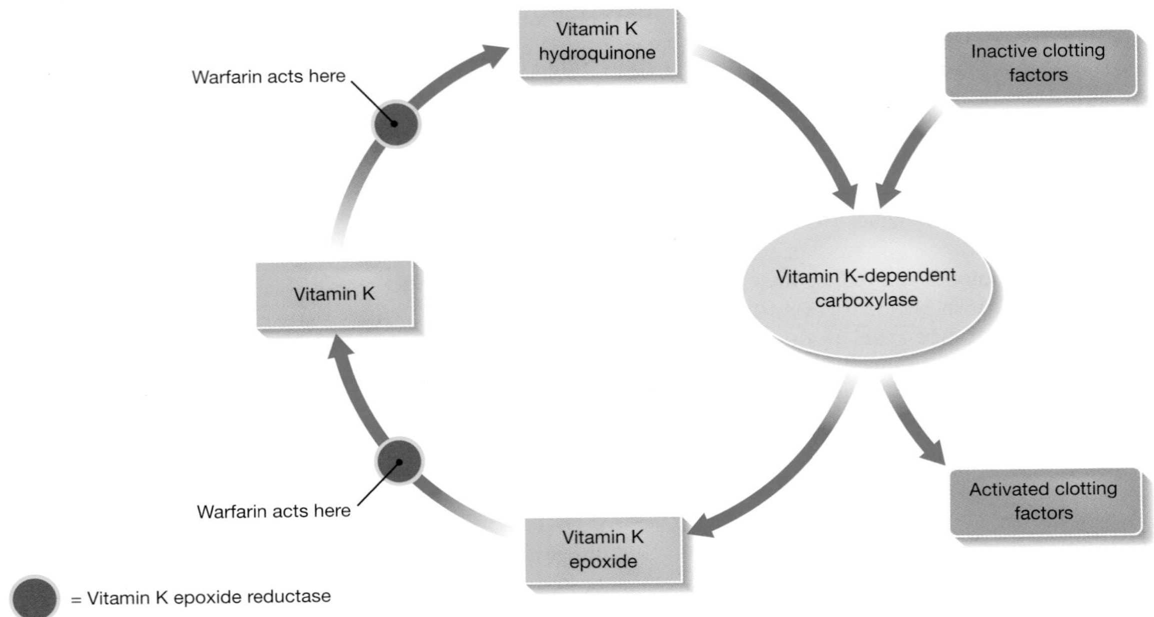


Figure 37.2 A diagram demonstrating the difference between unfractionated heparin and low molecular weight heparin

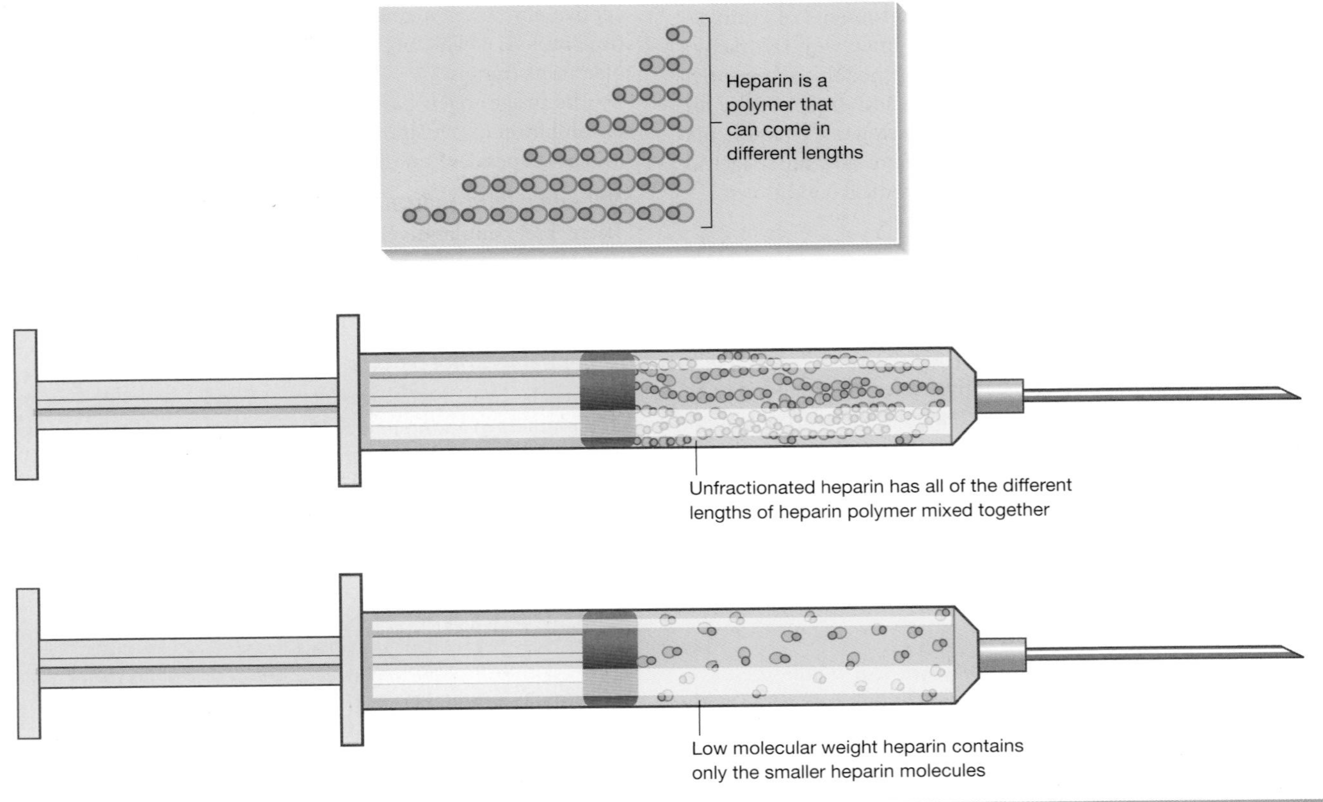


*Medicines Management for Nurses at a Glance*. First Edition. Simon Young and Ben Pitcher. © 2016 John Wiley & Sons, Ltd. Published 2016 by John Wiley & Sons, Ltd.
www.ataglanceseries.com/nursing/medicinesmanagement

Clotting is an important process within the body. It is integral to the facilitation of haemostasis and the maintenance of the integrity of the cardiovascular system. However, while clotting is important, if the blood clots too much or when it is not supposed to, it can have serious and potentially life-threatening consequences. If a clot (thrombus) forms in the blood, it can be carried by the flow of the blood until it reaches a vessel that it is too big to fit through; it may occlude this vessel and prevent blood from flowing through it. Whatever that blood vessel was supplying will now be starved of blood and oxygen. If the thrombus lodges in a coronary artery, it will cause a myocardial infarction (MI); if it occludes a vessel in the brain, it may cause a cerebrovascular accident (CVA).

Both anticoagulants and antiplatelet drugs (see Chapter 37) are often referred to in lay terms as 'blood thinners'. However, this is not an accurate description of their action. The term 'anticoagulant' refers to drugs that interfere with the clotting cascade, whereas antiplatelet drugs specifically prevent the aggregation of platelets.

## Anticoagulants and the clotting cascade

The clotting cascade has two branches, each with multiple stages. The cascade begins with the exposure of the blood to a stimulus. This may be tissue damage or exposure to some form of foreign body. This activates a clotting factor, which activates the next, which in turn activates the next, until eventually a stable clot is formed. Inhibition of the activation of one of these factors will halt the cascade and prevent clot formation.

### Coumarins

- Warfarin (see Figure 37.1).
- Acenocoumarol.

#### *Indications*

Warfarin is one of the oldest and most widely used anticoagulants. It is very effective in reducing the risk of thrombus formation and is used in patients who require ongoing treatment for chronic risk of thrombus.

#### *Pharmacodynamics*

The clotting cascade is a series of activations of clotting factors. The activation of these factors is dependent upon vitamin K, which is incorporated into the cascade by the enzyme, vitamin K epoxide reductase. Warfarin (and other coumarins) is a similar molecule to vitamin K and a competitive substrate for this enzyme. When the warfarin is bound to the enzyme, the vitamin K cannot be used to activate the clotting factors. Because the coumarins do not irreversibly bind to the enzyme, but simply interfere with the binding of vitamin K, they do not completely prevent clotting, but slow it down and reduce it. By increasing the relative concentrations of warfarin and vitamin K, you can titrate the impact of the anticoagulant on the patient.

#### *Pharmacokinetics*

Coumarins are administered orally.

#### *Notable contra-indications/cautions and warnings*

The action of warfarin can easily be affected by other drugs. This can increase or decrease the effectiveness of the drug and increase the risk of thrombus formation or bleeding. While interactions occur with many drugs, warfarin is notable for having many interactions including with over-the-counter drugs (aspirin and ibuprofen), herbal remedies (St. John's wort), food stuffs (cranberry juice) and alcohol.

#### *Side effects/ADRs*

The side effects of warfarin include increased bruising and risk of bleeding.

**Clinical pointers**

The dosing of coumarins is titrated to the desired effect. This is measured by the **international normalised ratio (INR)**. This is a representation of how long the blood of a patient takes to clot compared with an average patient. If a patient's INR is 2 then their blood takes twice as long to clot. If the INR is 3, it takes 3 times as long. If the INR is 0.75, then the patient's blood will clot quickly and more easily than normal. Depending on the patient's relative risk of thrombus, they will have a target INR (atrial fibrillation target INR 2.5; recurrent deep vein thrombosis target INR 3.5) The dose will then be titrated until the patient's INR hits the target. Should a patient be overdosed with warfarin, it is possible to reverse its action by administering vitamin K.

### Heparin

- Unfractionated heparin.
- Low molecular weight heparin.

#### *Indications*

An alternative to warfarin, heparin is more often used in acute circumstances such as treatment of an MI or prevention of deep vein thrombosis for patients following surgery.

#### *Pharmacodynamics*

As with many processes in the body, there is a mechanism to switch off the clotting cascade. Antithrombin inactivates two key factors, thrombin and factor X, and therefore halts the coagulation cascade preventing a clot from being formed. Heparin binds to antithrombin and increases its activity a thousand fold.

#### *Pharmacokinetics*

Heparin cannot be taken orally so it is administered intravenously or subcutaneously. It is a polymer that exists in different lengths. Unfractionated heparin is a mixture of all sizes, usually administered in hospital via infusion. Low molecular weight heparins are just the shorter polymers, usually administered subcutaneously via pre-filled syringes (see Figure 37.2).

#### *Notable contra-indications/cautions and warnings*

It is possible for patients to develop heparin-induced thrombocytopenia and thrombosis (HITT). This can cause a reduction in platelet count and reduced clotting.

#### *Side effects/ADRs*

The side effects of heparin include increased bruising and risk of bleeding, especially at the site of administration.

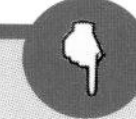

**Clinical pointers**

The effectiveness of heparin is measured via the activated partial thromboplastin time (APTT).

Should a patient be overdosed with heparin, it is possible to use protamine to reverse its action. Protamine binds to heparin, thereby inactivating it.

# Antiplatelet drugs

**Figure 38.1** An entry from an in-patient medication chart illustrating how some antiplatelet drugs might be prescribed and some key features to be considered when they are administered

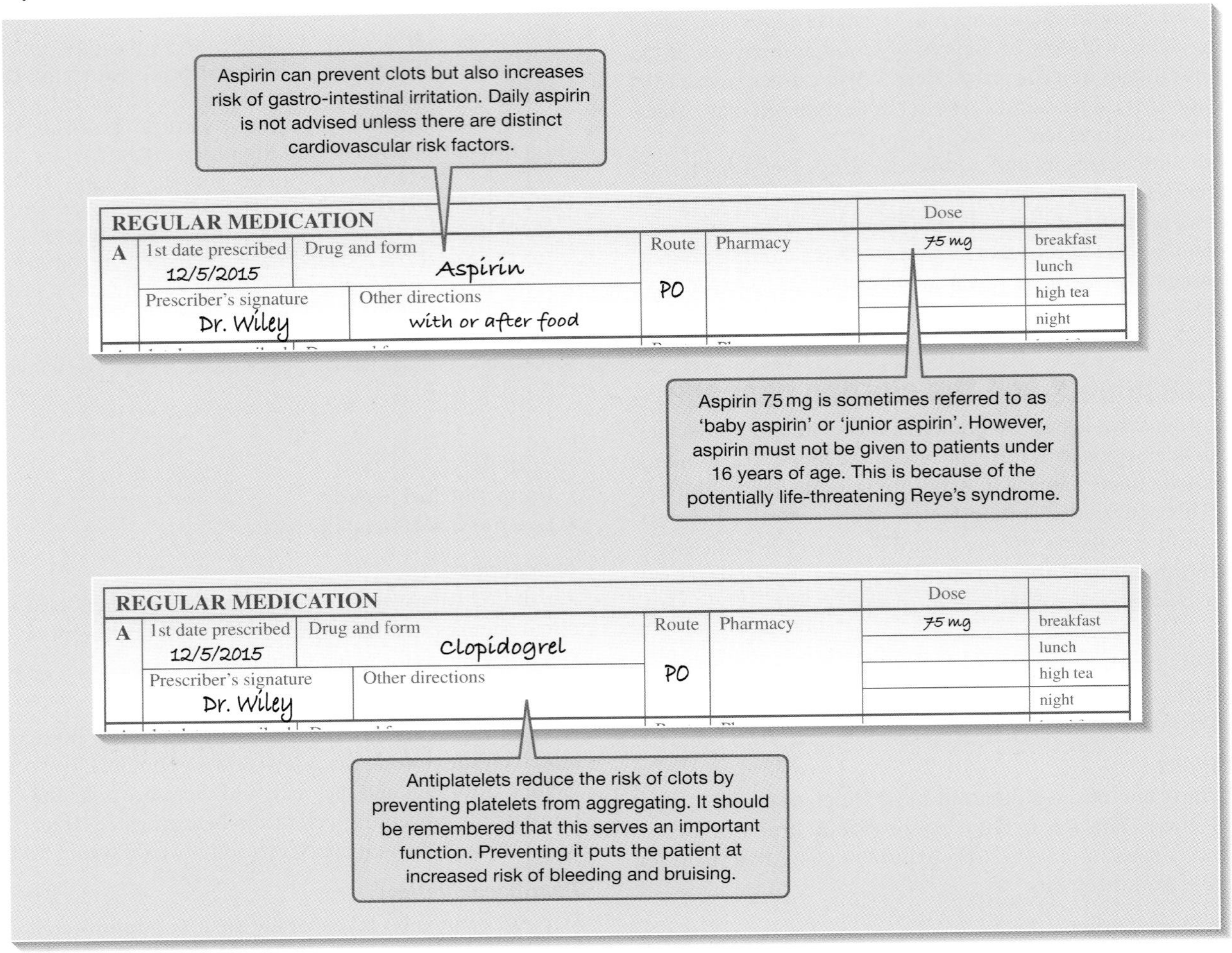

Antiplatelet drugs act directly on the platelets, preventing them from clumping together (aggregating). This is an effective way of preventing thrombus formation (Figure 38.1).

## Aspirin

Aspirin is widely used and well known for its anti-inflammatory and antipyretic properties. However, it is also widely used as an antiplatelet agent.

### Indications

Aspirin can be used in the secondary prevention of thrombotic cerebrovascular or cardiovascular disease. By preventing platelets from clumping together, it can prevent the formation of thrombi and thereby help prevent heart attacks and strokes.

Platelets (thrombocytes) play an important part in the formation of a clot. If the integrity of a blood vessel is compromised (by trauma or atherosclerosis), platelets come into contact with collagen or other tissue factors. This activates the platelet, changing its shape and allowing it to bind to other platelets. As more and more platelets bind together, they form a plug that in the case of trauma will block the outflow of blood from the vessel. In ill health, this plug can form a thrombus that may be carried along in the bloodstream until it lodges in a narrowing of the vessel, potentially causing a myocardial infarction (MI) or cerebrovascular accident (CVA).

### Pharmacodynamics

Normally, once the receptors on the outside of the platelet have been stimulated, an enzyme called cyclooxygenase-1 (COX-1) is activated. COX-1 facilitates the production of thromboxane, which in turn facilitates the activation of the platelet. Aspirin is a COX-1 inhibitor and therefore prevents the formation of thromboxane and the activation of the platelet.

### Pharmacokinetics

Aspirin is usually administered in tablet form and taken daily.

### Side effects/adverse drug reactions (ADRs)

Aspirin is a COX inhibitor and COX is responsible for the production of chemical mediators all over the body. This gives it a broad spectrum of activity but also a number of side effects. The most notable is the reduction in gastric mucous production and increase in gastric acid production. This combination can cause gastric irritation and even stomach ulcers. It is important that these side effects are not magnified by using aspirin with other drugs with similar mechanisms of action or side-effect profiles (particularly other non-steroidal anti-inflammatory drugs [NSAIDs] such as ibuprofen or naproxen).

**Clinical pointers**

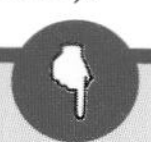

Aspirin tablets of varying strength can be bought from retailers. A single dose of aspirin for pain relief is typically 2 × 300 mg, while the daily dose as an antiplatelet drug is a single 75 mg tablet, sometimes referred to as a 'baby aspirin'. There have been accounts of patients mistakenly taking a single 300 mg tablet every day rather than the 75 mg dose. When taken daily for long periods of time, this larger dose can have a cumulative effect that can place the patient at greater risk of gastric irritation and ulcer formation.

## Clopidogrel (Plavix®)

### Indications

Clopidogrel is used to help prevent clots in patients with a high risk of having an MI or stroke (or given to those who have already had one). It is sometimes used in patients when warfarin is unsuitable.

### Pharmacodynamics

Clopidogrel binds to and blocks an adenosine diphosphate (ADP) receptor on the outside of a platelet. This prevents the platelet from becoming activated and prevents fibrin cross-linking, which will hold the clot together.

### Pharmacokinetics

Given in tablet form, clopidogrel is actually a prodrug. It needs to be activated by a liver enzyme before it can have any effect.

## Dipyridamole

### Indications

Dipyridamole is commonly used alongside other anticoagulant therapy to help prevent clots in high-risk patients, especially those with synthetic replacement heart valves.

### Pharmacodynamics

Cyclic adenosine monophosphate (cAMP) is a second messenger involved in many cellular processes. Dipyridamole inhibits the phosphodiesterase enzymes responsible for the breakdown of cAMP; the resultant increase in cAMP levels has widespread effects on a number of cellular activities. One effect is to reduce the activation and aggregation of platelets, preventing them from forming into a thrombus.

### Pharmacokinetics

Administered orally, dipiridamole is available as a slow-release oral formulation allowing consistent dosing over time from a single administration.

## Other antiplatelets and anticoagulants

### Fondaparinux

A newer drug, fondaparinux, is an alternative to heparin (more specifically, low molecular weight heparin). It inhibits an important part of the clotting cascade (Factor Xa). It is administered by subcutaneous injection.

### Dabigatran

A newer agent, which is a member of a group of drugs called novel oral anticoagulants (NOACs), dabigatran is used as an alternative to warfarin when warfarin is unsuitable or the patient has been unable to manage the complex dosing regimen. Dabigatran is a thrombin inhibitor administered as an oral tablet and does not need to be titrated according to the international normalised ratio (INR). This makes its management much easier, which improves concordance. However, it also makes it harder to assess whether it is acting effectively.

### Fibrinolytic drugs

If a thrombus does form, it can have potentially life-threatening outcomes. There are a range of drugs that can be administered to break down the clot (thrombolytics). These drugs generally work by transforming plasminogen into plasmin, which in turn breaks down fibrin, allowing the clot to dissipate. These drugs can prevent long-term damage by breaking down the problem thrombus. However, they will affect any clots in the body, including those that have been formed in response to trauma in order to prevent haemorrhage. As such, there is a significant risk of bleeding if a patient has any cuts or wounds.

# Musculoskeletal disorders

**Figure 39.1** An entry from an in-patient medication chart illustrating how allopurinol and indometacin may be prescribed and some key features to be considered when they are administered

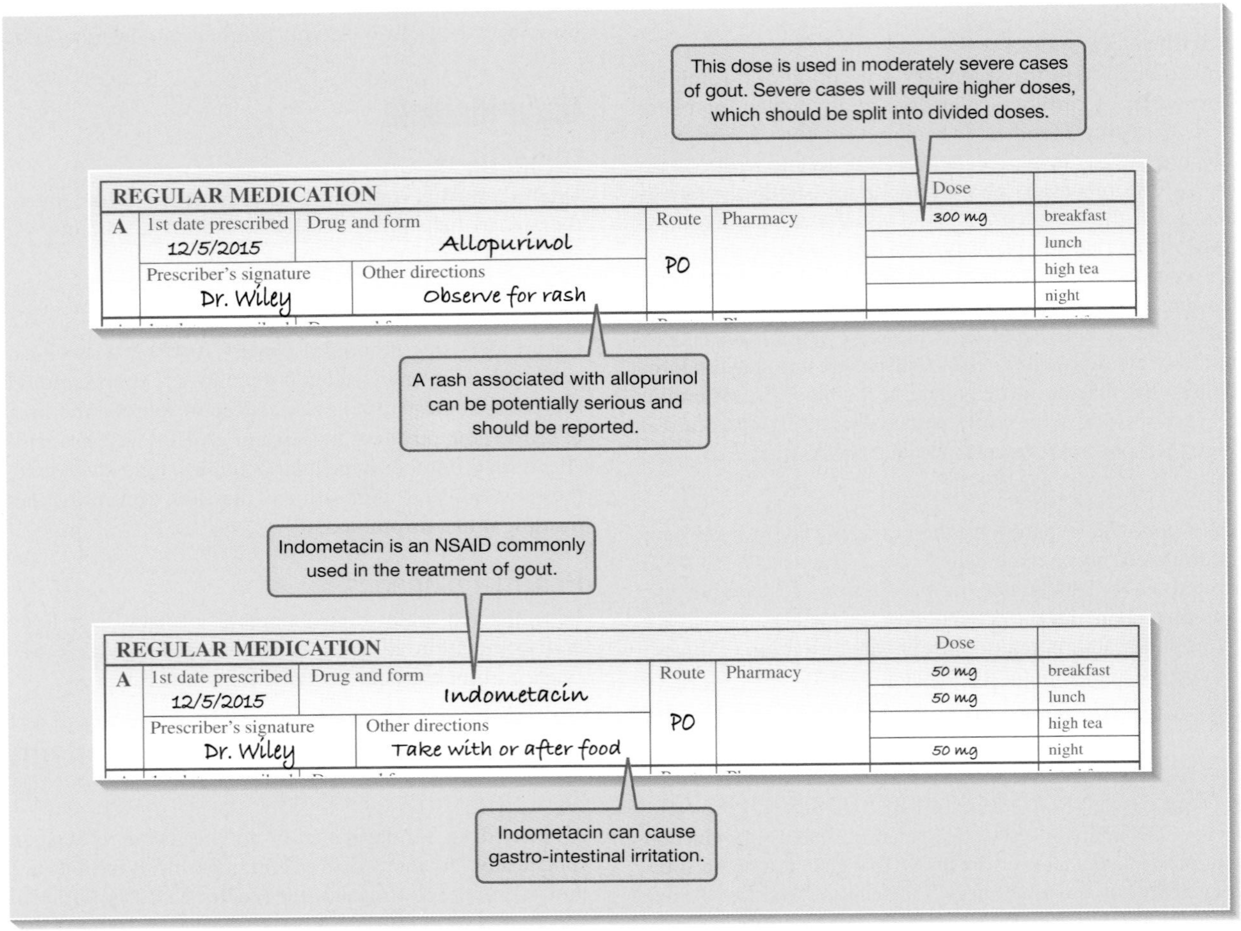

There are a range of conditions that affect the musculoskeletal system. These include conditions such as osteoporosis and rheumatoid arthritis. Each of these conditions has complex pharmacological interventions and management profiles. This chapter will consider some of the more commonly encountered interventions for musculoskeletal conditions (Figure 39.1).

Many of these disorders cause deterioration and pain in the joints. The pain and loss of mobility can have a severe impact on people's lives. Some of these disorders, such as osteoarthritis, are caused by the wear and tear of the joints through repeated use and injury. Rheumatoid arthritis occurs when the body's own immune system causes significant harmful inflammation of the joints.

Because most of these diseases involve pain and inflammation, their symptoms can be controlled with drugs such as opioid analgesics (Chapter 23), non-steroidal anti-inflammatory drugs (NSAIDs) (Chapter 40) or steroids (Chapter 14).

## Gout

Gout is a painful disorder in which increased levels of uric acid within the blood (hyperuricaemia) result in the formation of crystals within a patient's joints. This can cause extreme pain and inflammation. In popular culture, the cause of gout is often attributed to the excessive lifestyle of the rich; this is, however, a largely false perception. Gout can be exacerbated by lifestyle factors such as alcohol consumption, diet and medication. However, its underlying cause is either an over-production of uric acid or a reduced ability of the kidneys to remove uric acid from the blood. This can be hereditary and is often associated with other diseases such as psoriasis or renal failure. Gout can also occur as a result of certain drugs such as chemotherapy.

Pharmacological interventions for gout can be categorised according to their role of either controlling the condition or treating acute exacerbations.

## Allopurinol

### Indications

Allopurinol is the most commonly used pharmacological intervention for the prevention of gout.

### Pharmacodynamics

Uric acid is an end product of a variety of metabolic pathways in which the enzyme xanthine oxidase plays an important role. Allopurinol is a xanthine oxidase inhibitor and therefore prevents the formation of uric acid and reduces its levels within the blood.

### Pharmacokinetics

Allopurinol is only administered in tablet form, usually with food.

### Side effects/adverse drug reactions (ADRs)

Allopurinol can cause hypersensitivity reactions in some patients. If a patient develops a rash, allopurinol should be discontinued.

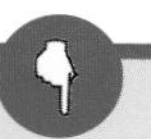

**Clinical pointers**

Allopurinol is used as a prophylactic to prevent attacks of gout. It is not meant to be used to help treat an acute attack of gout: in fact, it is believed that using allopurinol may exacerbate an existing attack.

## Colchicine

### Indications

Colchicine is prescribed to try and relieve the symptoms of a gout attack in progress.

### Pharmacodynamics

Colchicine is primarily an antimitotic drug that prevents cellular replication. However, the exact mechanism of action of colchicine in treating gout is not fully understood. It appears to inhibit the migration of neutrophils (a type of white blood cell) to the affected joint. This reduces the amount of inflammation.

### Pharmacokinetics

An initial dose of 1 mg is given followed by subsequent doses of 500 micrograms to a maximum dose of 6 mg (or until the symptoms are resolved).

### Notable contra-indications/cautions and warnings

Colchicine is a cytotoxic drug that should be absolutely avoided in pregnant women because of the risk of teratogenesis.

### Side effects/ADRs

Colchicine is a potentially toxic drug with unpleasant side effects and a narrow therapeutic window. Side effects include nausea and vomiting that can often be severe and may prevent the patient from completing the course of treatment. Because of the narrow therapeutic window, it is easy to overdose on colchicine.

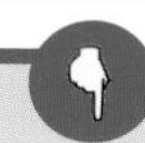

**Clinical pointers**

There are a number of folk remedies for the prevention of gout, although patient surveys report that the best means of prevention is through dietary control and increased intake of water (which appears to help dilute the level of uric acid in the blood and help its clearance from the body). However, there are pharmacological options.

#### *Cod liver oil and glucosamine*

There are a number of over-the-counter supplements popular with patients for the prevention and treatment of joint conditions. There are varying amounts of evidence to support the use of some of these agents.

**Cod liver oil** People often compare the action of cod liver oil on joints to adding oil to a creaking hinge. However, this is an incomplete explanation. As discussed in Chapter 40, prostaglandins are inflammatory mediators that are produced by the conversion of arachidonic acid by cyclooxygenase (COX). NSAIDs work by inhibiting COX, reducing the production of prostaglandins. Cod liver oil provides a supply of eicosapentaenoic acid, which is a competitive substrate for the COX enzyme. Essentially, the COX enzyme is flooded with the alternative substrate. This means that it can bind to less arachadonic acid and produce fewer prostaglandins. This results in less inflammation. Cod liver oil is a rich source of vitamin A, which should be avoided by pregnant women.

**Glucosamine** Glucosamine and other similar agents (such as chondroitin) provide the body with excess amounts of the raw materials required to produce cartilage and synovial fluid. There have been a number of studies that have identified that glucosamine may reduce pain and improve function of joints beyond a placebo effect.

# Non-steroidal anti-inflammatory drugs and non-opioid analgesics

**Figure 40.1** An entry from an in-patient medication chart illustrating how paracetamol and NSAIDs may be prescribed and some key features to be considered when they are administered

Packets of paracetamol often state that you can take 2 tablets (2 x 500 mg) every 4 hours. This is true. However, there is a maximum dose of 4 g in 24 hours. Doses should be spaced 6-hourly to avoid accidental overdosing.

| REGULAR MEDICATION | | | | | Dose | |
|---|---|---|---|---|---|---|
| A | 1st date prescribed 12/5/2015 | Drug and form Paracetamol 500 mg tablets | Route PO | Pharmacy | 1 g | breakfast |
| | | | | | 1 g | lunch |
| | Prescriber's signature Dr. Wiley | Other directions | | | 1 g | high tea |
| | | | | | 1 g | night |
| A | 1st date prescribed 12/5/2015 | Drug and form Naproxen | Route PO | Pharmacy | 250 mg | breakfast |
| | | | | | 250 mg | lunch |
| | Prescriber's signature Dr. Wiley | Other directions Take with food | | | 250 mg | high tea |
| | | | | | 250 mg | night |

NSAIDs can cause gastric irritation. Taking them with food can help reduce the risk of damage. In some cases proton pump inhibitors may be prescribed alongside NSAIDs to further reduce risk. NSAIDs are contra-indicated in patients who have a history of gastric ulcers.

*Medicines Management for Nurses at a Glance*. First Edition. Simon Young and Ben Pitcher. © 2016 John Wiley & Sons, Ltd. Published 2016 by John Wiley & Sons, Ltd.
www.ataglanceseries.com/nursing/medicinesmanagement

# Non-steroidal anti-inflammatory drugs

## Indications

Inflammation is a natural part of the healing process triggered by a damaging stimulus such as physical trauma or infection. In other diseases (such as auto-immune disorders), inflammation can run amok and cause damage to otherwise healthy tissues. Regardless of the cause, inflammation is painful and pharmacological options have been developed to manage it (Figure 40.1). One treatment involves the non-steroidal anti-inflammatory drugs (NSAIDs). They are named as such because they are an alternative to steroids (Chapter 14).

## Pharmacodynamics

Inflammation is controlled by a group of chemical mediators called prostaglandins. Some prostaglandins are produced at all times and perform various other functions around the body. Others are induced in response to trauma and trigger physiological responses such as vasodilation (causing redness and warmth), increased tissue permeability (causing swelling) and pain.

Prostaglandins are synthesised by two enzymes: cyclooxygenase-1 (COX-1) and cyclooxygenase-2 (COX-2). NSAIDs act by inhibiting these enzymes and thereby preventing the production of prostaglandins and subsequent inflammation. The COX-1 enzyme is present at all times and synthesises the prostaglandins responsible for various housekeeping functions, while the COX-2 enzyme is induced in response to trauma and produces the prostaglandins associated with inflammation.

## Pharmacokinetics

NSAIDs are primarily administered orally in tablet form. However, they can also be administered as suppositories or topical preparations.

## Side effects/adverse drug reactions (ADRs)

As discussed earlier, prostaglandins play a role in inflammation but also serve a variety of housekeeping functions within the body. The disruption of these functions is responsible for the major side effects of these drugs. One of the most notable functions is to stimulate the production of protective gastric mucus and reduce the secretion of gastric acid. If this action is disrupted, it can cause gastric irritation and even gastric ulcers. It is important, therefore, that NSAIDs are avoided in patients with a history of gastric ulcers.

It was theorised that, if a drug could be devised that only inhibited COX-2, it would be possible to produce an anti-inflammatory drug without side effects. Selective COX-2 inhibitors were developed, but it was soon discovered that inhibiting COX-2 increased cardiovascular risk and many of them were withdrawn from the market (although parecoxib and etoricoxib still remain in use).

Most NSAIDs inhibit both COX-1 and COX-2 enzymes to various degrees and therefore cause some gastric irritation and increase cardiovascular risk. Gastric irritation can be mitigated by taking the drug with food or using other drugs to control gastric acid secretion. Cardiovascular risk is present but is less than the risk caused by inactivity in chronic pain conditions such as rheumatoid arthritis. Other side effects can include nephrotoxicity and increased risk of bleeding.

# Details of common NSAIDs

**Aspirin** (acetylsalicylic acid) is one of the oldest and weakest of the NSAIDs. It has a broad range of uses, acting as an anti-inflammatory, analgesic, antipyretic and antiplatelet agent. Aspirin should not be given to children (16 years old or younger) because of the rare but potentially fatal Reye's syndrome.

**Ibuprofen** has greater COX-2 specificity than aspirin and is associated with a more potent anti-inflammatory effect and fewer gastro-intestinal side effects. It is available without prescription; however, in chronic conditions it may be prescribed at much higher doses than available over the counter.

**Diclofenac** has a stronger anti-inflammatory and analgesic action than ibuprofen but also more severe side effects. It is available in a range of dosage forms. It has largely been superseded by other NSAIDs with milder side effects.

**Naproxen** has a stronger anti-inflammatory and analgesic action than ibuprofen but it has lower cardiovascular risk associated with it. It does, however, cause significant gastric irritation.

**Indometacin** is a powerful NSAID often used to treat severe inflammation caused by diseases such as rheumatoid arthritis. Its strength is accompanied by more severe side effects.

# Non-opioid analgesics

## Indications

Paracetamol is one of the most commonly used drugs for the control of mild to moderate pain and pyrexia. However, unlike NSAIDs, it has very limited anti-inflammatory action and few side effects. It is commonly used in hospital environments and at home. It is available without prescription and can be bought from pharmacies and shops.

## Pharmacodynamics

The exact mechanism of action of paracetamol is not fully understood. While it is believed to be a COX inhibitor, it demonstrates neither the gastric irritation of a COX-1 inhibitor nor the anti-inflammatory action and cardiovascular risk profile of a COX-2 inhibitor. Theories about its mechanism of action include inhibition of other subvariants of COX or attributing its effect to entirely different mechanisms such as the endogenous cannabinoid system.

## Pharmacokinetics

Paracetamol is normally administered orally. However, it undergoes some first-pass metabolism in the liver. The same dose of paracetamol will have a greater effect if administered intravenously.

## Notable contra-indications/cautions and warnings

Side effects for paracetamol are relatively uncommon. In fact, paracetamol is a very safe drug, as long as it is taken within the recommended dosing limits. However, if there is an overdose, it can cause critical damage to the liver. This occurs because one of the mechanisms for metabolising paracetamol produces a toxic intermediate that is immediately neutralised by glutathione. The problem is that the body has a limited supply of glutathione, which will be depleted if someone consumes too much paracetamol. Once it runs out, the toxic intermediate will no longer be neutralised and will damage the cells of the liver. The treatment for paracetamol overdose is intravenous acetylcysteine, which the body then converts into glutathione.

# 41 Topical agents and emollients

**Figure 41.1** Single fingertip unit (FTU) – the quantity of cream that is squeezed onto a patient's fingertip from the crease of the first knuckle to the tip of the finger

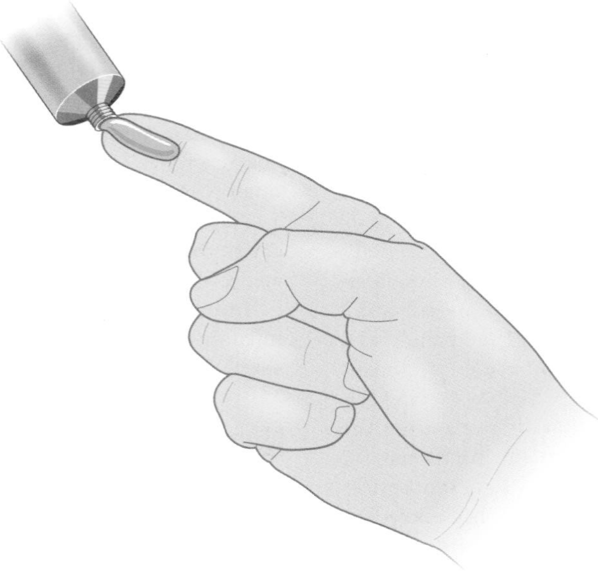

**Figure 41.2** The number of FTUs that might be used to cover various regions of the body

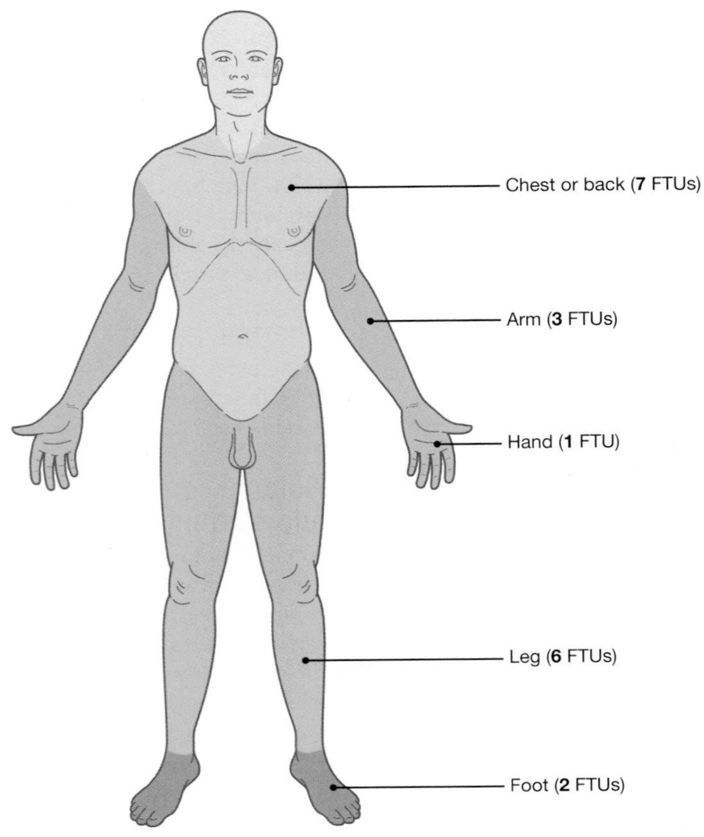


*Medicines Management for Nurses at a Glance*. First Edition. Simon Young and Ben Pitcher. © 2016 John Wiley & Sons, Ltd. Published 2016 by John Wiley & Sons, Ltd.
www.ataglanceseries.com/nursing/medicinesmanagement

While not always considered as 'serious' as other medical problems, dermatological conditions can cause significant discomfort and pain to patients, affect body image and result in hospitalisation. Skin complaints may be part of an underlying chronic disorder, but it is important to remember that they may also be part of an allergic or adverse reaction that may need to be properly assessed.

Not all treatments used in dermatology are applied directly to the skin but a large proportion are. This topical administration is advantageous in this case because it allows one to apply the medication directly to the target area, thereby achieving a local effect with minimal scope for systemic side effects. However, topical administration does introduce some difficulties, particularly how to regulate dosing. Unlike other routes of administration, it is difficult to measure out exact quantities and it is even more important to take into account the size of the individual and therefore the area of skin that needs to be covered. There are strategies to deal with this though.

## Fingertip units

A fingertip unit (FTU) is the quantity of cream that is squeezed onto a patient's fingertip from the crease of the first knuckle to the tip of the finger (Figure 41.1). Because people are different sizes, the amount of cream required to cover a given part of the body (e.g. leg) will vary. However, there will be a general correlation between the size of a person's leg and the size of their fingertip. Therefore, we can use FTUs to guide us on how much cream should be applied to an area of the body to provide appropriate dosing whatever the size of the patient (Figure 41.2).

## Emollients

There are a variety of skin conditions, such as eczema and psoriasis that result in the skin drying and scaling. This can cause discomfort and presents a risk of infection. An emollient is a product that occludes the skin's surface to prevent loss of moisture. This is generally achieved by applying some form of oil to the skin. Historically, animal or vegetable oils were used (and in some cases still are today); however, most emollients now use some form of petroleum derivative, such as paraffin wax.

The term 'emollient' is essentially another word for 'moisturiser'. However, most of what are referred to as moisturisers (used in cosmetics or in general skin care) have added ingredients, such as fragrances, which can cause irritation and may actually dry the skin out. As a result, the term 'emollient' is usually used in reference products used to treat a skin condition, whereas 'moisturiser' is used more in the context of general skin care.

### Application

When used in the treatment of chronic conditions such as eczema and psoriasis, emollients need to be applied regularly and in large quantities. The amount applied varies from product to product; however, because there are no pharmacologically active ingredients in emollients, it is not really possible to overdose and there is greater risk in under-treating than over-treating. It is commonly recommended to apply emollients at least 3 or 4 times a day. They should be applied to the skin in the direction of hair growth (i.e. from the top of the arm down towards the hand or from the knee down towards the foot) to reduce the risk of developing folliculitis.

### Keeping it clean

Because of the large quantities of emollient that are administered, it is not supplied in a tube but in a tub or 'pump dispenser'. While the tub makes it easier to access the emollient, it presents a potential hazard. If the patient (or healthcare professional) puts their hand into the tub, they introduce bacteria into the emollient. The bacteria can grow and multiply there, and it is therefore possible to inadvertently spread bacteria around the patient and infect broken skin. To help prevent this, emollients should be removed from the tub using a clean spoon or spatula before being applied to the patient.

Emollients are generally categorised as creams or ointments. While they have the same key ingredients, ointments contain a greater proportion of oil, making them more effective in occluding the surface of the skin. However, this also makes them less palatable to patients because they leave the skin feeling greasy and worsen other skin conditions such as acne or folliculitis. Creams are less oily and feel like they are absorbed more easily, leaving the skin dry and avoiding some of those unpleasant after-effects. While technically less effective, patients are more likely to follow the treatment plan if they are happier with the product, and this will probably result in a more effective treatment of the condition.

### Added ingredients

While the primary ingredient of emollients is oil or wax, some products include additional additives to augment their action. Urea (which is commonly present on the skin as a component of sweat) is added to some products to help soften keratin. This is particularly useful in conditions that produce hard scaly patches of skin. It has been mentioned that some skin conditions can cause breaks in the skin that leave the patient at risk of infection. To help combat this, there are some emollients that have an antimicrobial agent added.

### Washing products

Regular soap can dry out the skin and exacerbate eczema. Therefore, patients are often recommended to avoid soap-based products and to use the variety of emollient bath and shower preparations that are available.

# Topical steroids

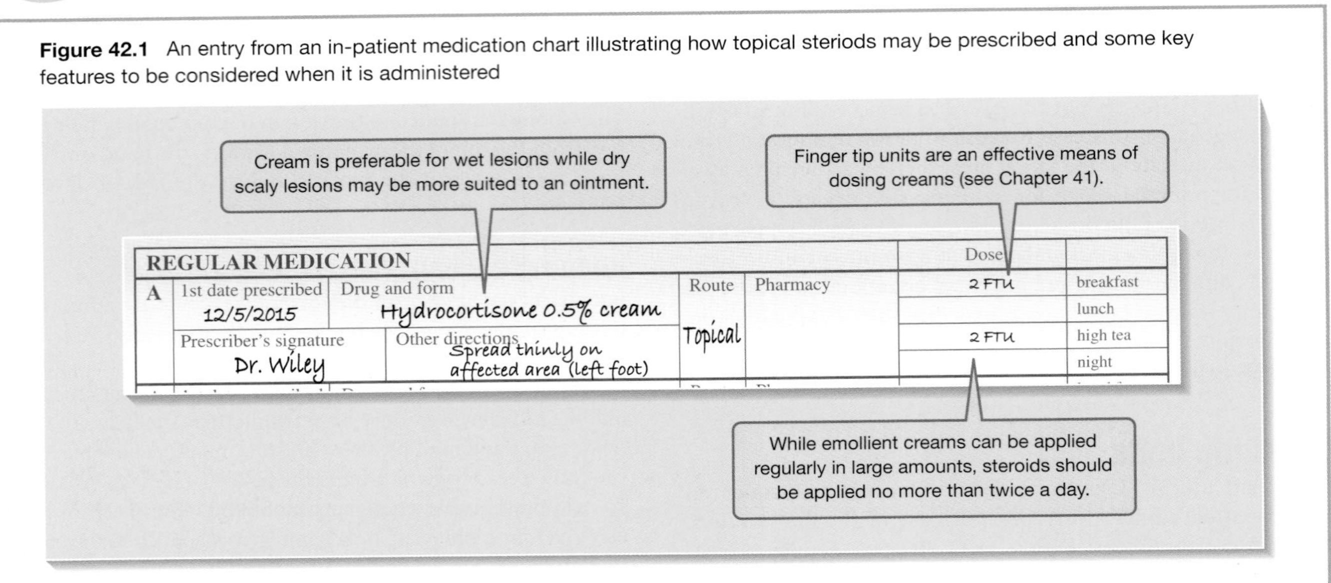


**Figure 42.1** An entry from an in-patient medication chart illustrating how topical steriods may be prescribed and some key features to be considered when it is administered

Many skin conditions (such as eczema) are either caused by or involve inflammatory processes. As discussed in Chapter 14, steroids are powerful anti-inflammatory agents. Steroid creams come in a variety of strengths that are selected depending on the seriousness of the condition (Figure 42.1).

## Commonly used steroid creams

- Hydrocortisone.
- Clobetasone (Eumovate®).
- Betamethasone (Betnovate®).
- Beclometasone.
- Clobetasol (Dermovate®).

## Pharmacodynamics

Topical steroids have the same pharmacodynamics as steroids taken by any other route. They stimulate the production of lipocortin-1, which inhibits phospholipase, an enzyme that plays a key role in producing inflammatory mediators. With this enzyme inhibited, the inflammatory mediators are not produced and the inflammation is reduced.

## Pharmacokinetics

Topical steroids are applied directly to the affected area of skin, the intention being to achieve a local effect without causing the systemic side effects associated with oral or intravenous administration. However, systemic effects have occasionally been noted in patients using the stronger varieties of topical steroid.

Topical steroids are available in a variety of formulations:

- Creams are more water based and are suitable for application to skin that is broken and moist.
- Ointments contain more oil and are useful in treating dry or scaly skin.
- Lotions are effective in treating areas where there is a lot of hair, such as the scalp.

## Side effects/adverse drug reactions (ADRs)

Because the cream is applied locally, most of the side effects seen are at or around the site of application. The local action of the steroid can cause a thinning of the skin, irritation and increased hair growth. Steroids are immunosuppressants so, if the affected skin is infected, the topical steroid may slow healing and allow the infection to spread.

While emollients can be applied in large quantities without worrying about overdose, topical steroids should be applied in moderation. This is especially true of the stronger formulations that can cause systemic side effects such as adrenal suppression. Because of this, the lowest strength of steroid that is still fully effective should be used. The most potent steroid creams should only be used when directed by a specialist.

However, it is important to remember that the side-effect profile of topical steroids is quite mild. Patients may need to be reassured of this because the impact of the side effects of these agents is far less than the impact of under-treating the eczema; however, fear of side effects is a leading cause of non-compliance.

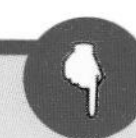

### Clinical pointers

The British National Formulary (BNF) organises topical steroids into categories of potency. The mildest can be bought over the counter without prescription, while the most potent are only recommended for short-term use under specialist supervision:

- **Mild** (e.g. hydrocortisone).
- **Moderately potent** (e.g. betametasone [Betnovate-RD®], clobetasone [Eumovate®]).
- **Potent** (e.g. beclometasone).
- **Very potent** (e.g. clobetasol [Dermovate®]).

Topical steroid containers will note the concentration of the drug expressed as a percentage.

While a higher percentage of a drug does mean a stronger preparation, it is important to remember that the difference of strength between mild and moderately potent steroids is great. As such, a moderately potent steroid with a smaller percentage concentration may be more effective than a mild steroid with a high percentage concentration (i.e. 1% hydrocortisone is considered milder than 0.05% clobetasone).

Different strengths of topical steroid are required depending on the severity of the condition being treated and the location on the body. Stronger steroids are required to treat areas of the body that have thicker skin, such as the soles of the feet. Areas of the body with thinner skin, such as the face or groin require weaker steroids.

## Topical steroids combined with antimicrobial agents

Conditions such as eczema, which can cause breaks in the integrity of the skin, can lead to infection. This can be bacterial, fungal and even viral – such as eczema herpeticum (herpes simplex) – which is considered a dermatological emergency. Infected eczemas often present as wet broken areas with weeping pus or a golden crust.

In severe infections, antibiotics are administered systemically. However, some topical steroids combined with antimicrobial agents are available that can help eliminate an infection or prevent it from spreading:

- Hydrocortisone with miconazole (Daktacort®).
- Hydrocortisone with clotrimazole (Canestan – HC®).

If an infection is suspected, ointments are often recommended rather than creams.

## Treatments for psoriasis

Psoriasis can appear to be a similar condition to eczema but has distinct process involved and therefore different treatments available. It is caused by an over-production of skin cells that present as plaques or pustules on the surface of the skin and can be itchy, painful and disfiguring. While emollients and topical steroids do form part of the management strategy for psoriasis, there are a number of treatments that are specifically intended for this condition.

Skin lotions and shampoos containing tar have proved very popular with patients who have psoriasis. However, there is limited evidence to support their use. They also tend to smell strongly and are not always appealing for patients to use.

Dithranol disrupts the ability of mitochondria to provide energy to a cell, which has the effect of slowing energy-dependent processes within the cell, such as cell division. This appears to prevent the excessive production of skin cells that cause psoriatic plaques. Dithranol tends to stain the skin (and clothing) brown, which can make it unappealing to patients.

Vitamin D (and analogues):

- Calcipotriol.
- Calcitriol.
- Acalcitol.

These drugs are commonly used in the treatment of osteoporosis. They are vitamin D analogues that help control the availability of calcium. However, they have been found to be effective in the treatment of psoriasis when applied topically. The mechanism of action is not fully understood but it is believed that the drugs modulate the ability of the cells to proliferate and therefore prevent the development of plaques. Unlike dithranol and tar-based treatments, vitamin D analogues have no accompanying smell and cause no staining, making them more popular with patients.

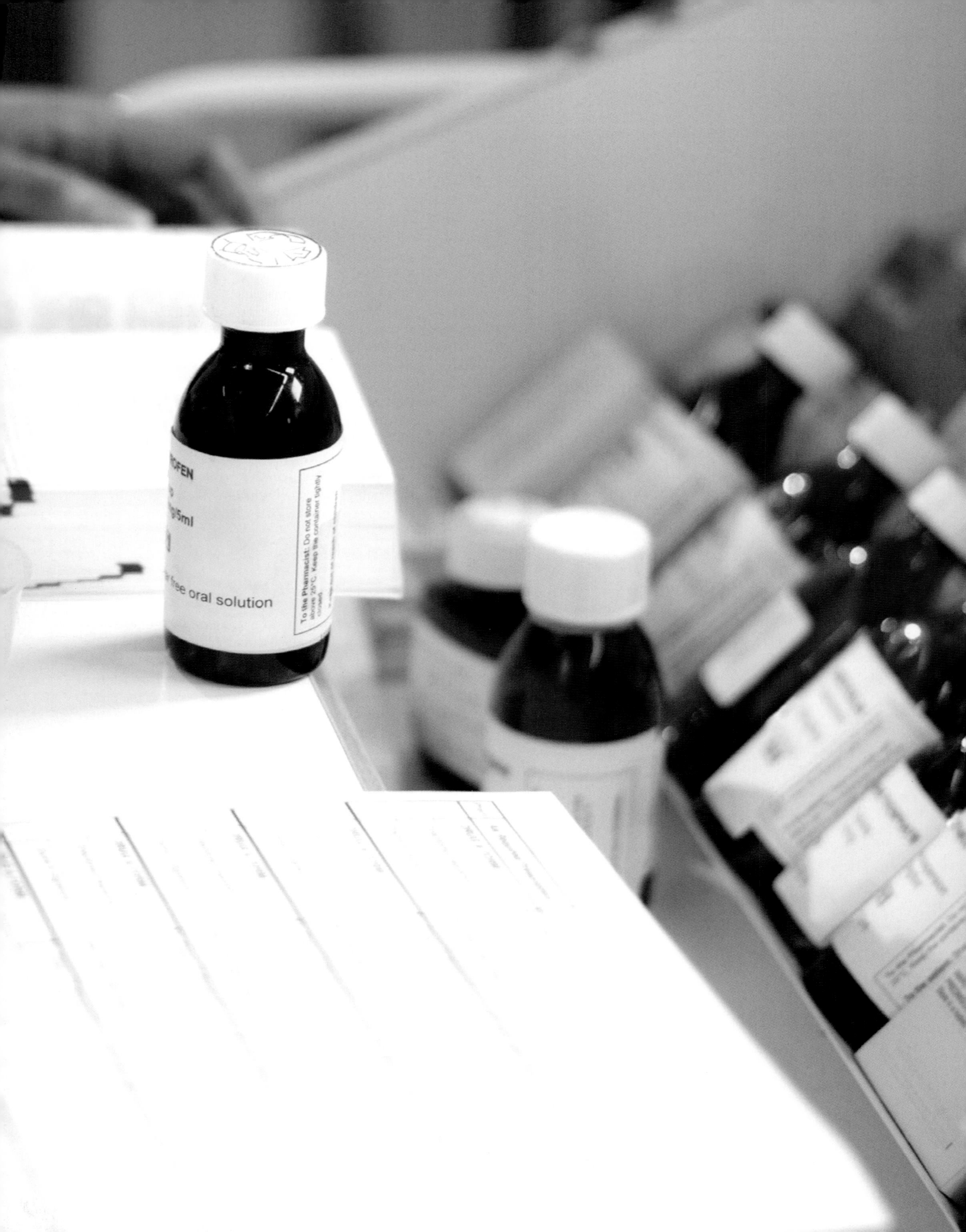
free oral solution
To the Pharmacist: Do not store
above 25°C. Keep the container tightly

# Safe and effective medicines management

Chapters

# 43 Medicines management in pregnancy and breastfeeding

**Figure 43.1** Entries from in-patient medication charts illustrating examples of medication that can impact upon a pregnant or breastfeeding woman

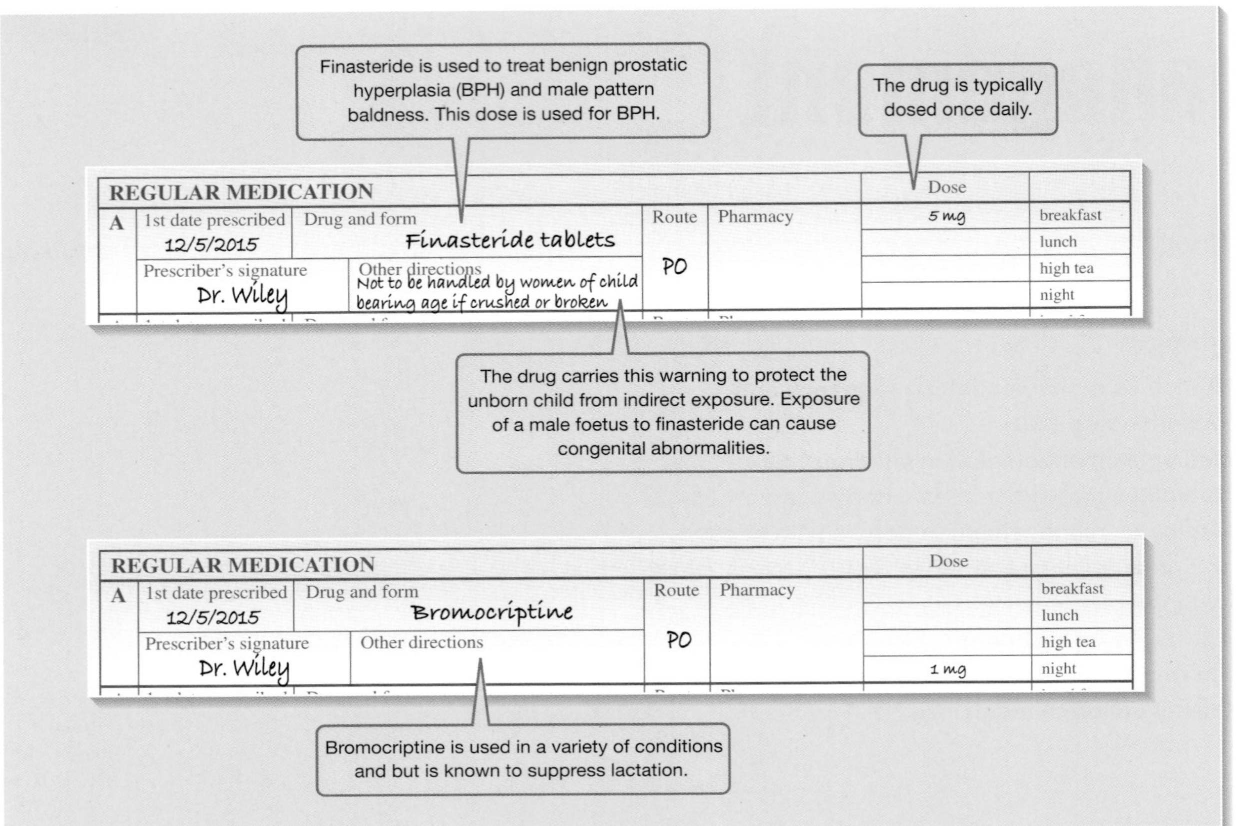


**Figure 43.2** An illustration of the effects of medication on the health and well-being of the foetus and mother through the stages of gestational development. The figure illustrates that medication taken during the gestational period can influence the child's development after birth (breastfeeding and the milestones attained in childhood)

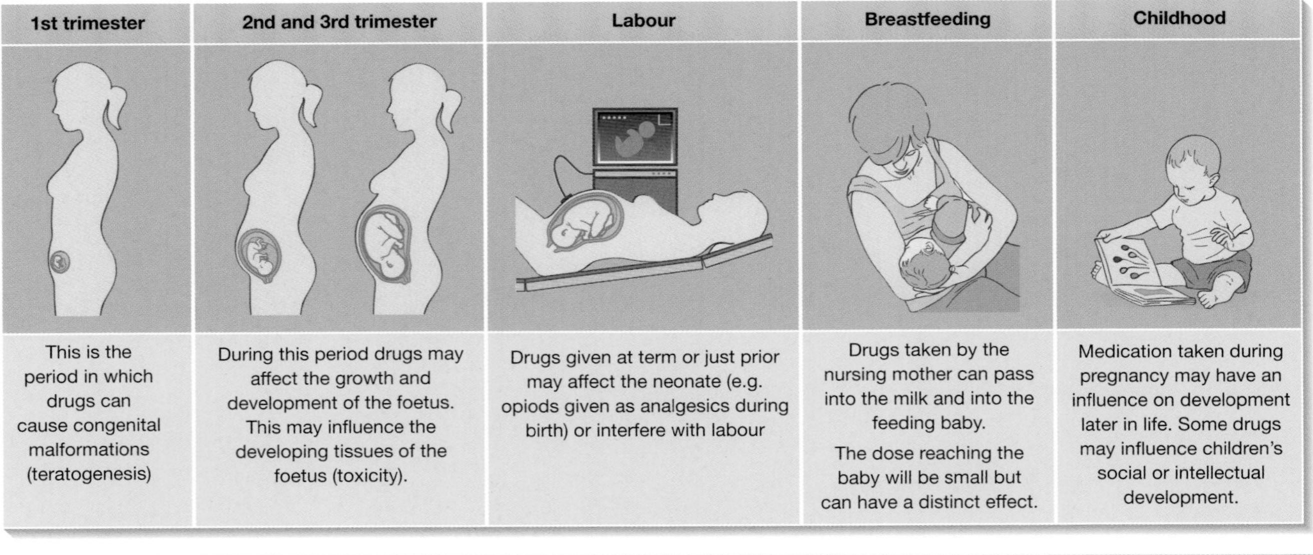

Drugs are essentially chemicals that have been designed to interact with the physiological systems of the body and evoke a change. That change typically serves to restore a balance that has been disturbed by a disease process. Selecting drugs in pregnancy is particularly complex. Not only do the needs of the patient (mother-to-be) need to be considered but also the needs of the foetus and, dependent on the stage of pregnancy, the process of giving birth (Figure 43.2).

The ill-considered use of the drug thalidomide in pregnant women in the late 1950s and early 1960s demonstrated a clear link between the use of medication and its potential to harm the foetus. As a consequence of the thalidomide tragedy, the way medicines are monitored when on the market and the approach to prescribing for pregnant women have improved significantly.

## General principles to using medicines in pregnancy

**Where possible, medicines should not be used during pregnancy**. Non-pharmacological interventions should always be considered first. This is not always an option: mothers with chronic conditions such as epilepsy, diabetes or hypertension may need medication throughout their pregnancy to maintain their health and that of the foetus.

**Where possible, drugs should be avoided during the first trimester of pregnancy**. The use of certain drugs during this stage of pregnancy may lead to congenital malformations (teratogenisis). This is challenging, because many patients will take drugs (both medicinal and recreational) before they are aware that they are pregnant.

**When drugs need to be used during pregnancy, those with established safety profiles should be used.** Pregnancy is a less suitable time for using black triangle agents (▼) or newer agents that have spent little time on the market (see Chapter 49). The testing of medicines on pregnant women is unethical so manufacturers have little or no data supporting medication use. If medication is used, as with other areas of medicines management practice, the lowest possible dose should be used for the shortest duration of time. The risk–benefit analysis performed by prescribers during pregnancy will be more complex. If women fear that a drug may harm their developing child, they may become non-adherent, and this becomes an important consideration in monitoring and assessing the progress of drug therapy.

**Always seek specialist advice when managing medicines in pregnant women**. The British National Formulary (BNF) has fairly comprehensive practical guidance; more detailed guidance can be found from specialists in their relevant fields. For example, neurologists will have some experience of managing epilepsy in pregnant females alongside their obstetric colleagues and midwives. Specialist texts such as *Drugs in Pregnancy and Lactation* (http://www.amazon.com/Drugs-Pregnancy-Lactation-Reference-Neonatal/dp/1608317080, last accessed 6 August, 2015) give further advice, and very specific specialist advice can be obtained from the UK Teratology Information Service.

Some texts will use the convention of the pre-embryonic stage (the first 17 days post-conception), the embryonic stage (typically days 18–56) and the foetal stage (weeks 8–38), rather than the trimester staging; this may better reflect the timing of processes such as implantation, when organ and tissue systems are formed, and the stages of maturation of the foetus in preparation for delivery.

## General approaches to using medicines during breastfeeding

Breastfeeding is the healthiest and most beneficial way of providing nutrients to an infant. The benefits of breastfeeding are well documented and the current campaigns that support and promote breastfeeding are an important part of developing the health and well-being of a child.

As with pregnancy, there is a shortage of evidence available on what impact medication that passes into breast milk has on a feeding child. In general, there are groups of drugs that are regarded as safe in breastfeeding. With regard to 'safe' drugs, the dose the infant receives is a small percentage of the dose taken by the mother. This small dose has little or no discernible effect on the feeding infant. Some caution should be exercised if the mother is taking a high dose or the child is more susceptible to the effect of the drug (e.g. the child has renal or hepatic impairment or was born prematurely). Hypersensitivity and allergic reactions can also occur in an infant who may be exposed to medication through breastfeeding.

Some drugs do pass in sufficient quantity into breast milk and hence into the infant. The BNF and the summary of product characteristics (SPC) of the relevant drug agent will give details of any concerns that may arise. The BNF highlights drugs that are to be used with caution or that are contra-indicated in breast feeding. Some drugs that affect the central nervous system may make an infant drowsy and they may have difficulty suckling as a consequence; some drugs can affect breast tenderness and milk production, and this may present in the course of caring for the woman and child. Please remember that a lack of evidence for using a drug when breastfeeding does not mean it is necessarily safe.

### Clinical pointers

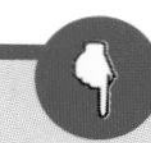

If you care for women of child-bearing age, mothers-to-be, or mothers and infants in the context of your practice, you must be aware of the medications that are regularly prescribed in that clinical arena, and of their potential impact on pregnant and breastfeeding patients and staff (Figure 43.1).

# 44 Medicines management in children

**Figure 44.1** Some considerations for using medications in children

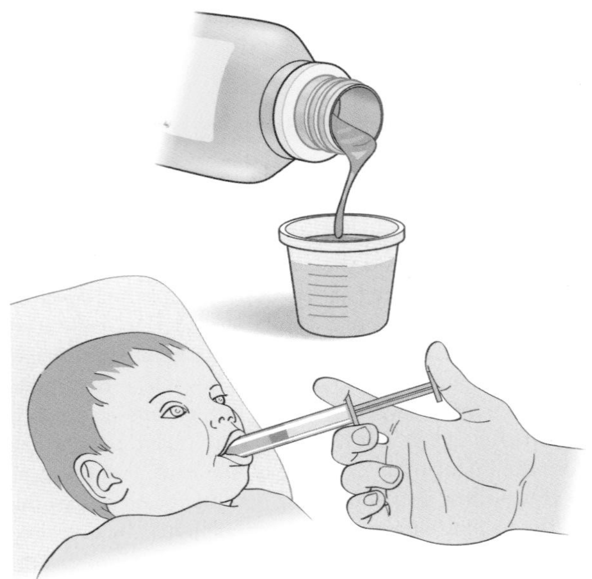

- Children will often find liquid medicines more acceptable than tablets but this may not always be the case. Ask the child or their parent or guardian about their preferences
- Not all liquid medicines are suitable for use in children – some contain unsuitable excipients such as sugar or alcohol
- Syrups and oral solutions may come in different strengths designed for children of different ages. It is important to use the correct strength to avoid accidental over- or under-dosing
- Oral syringes are often used when the volume to be administered is less than 5 ml or includes volumes of less than 5 ml
- Children's medicines should not be hidden in food or milk, unless specifically stated in the manufacturer's instructions. The foodstuff may combine with the medication rendering it ineffective. The medicine may make the foodstuff unpalatable

**Figure 44.2** A typical label for a medicine (in this case paracetamol prescribed for a child)

KEEP OUT OF THE REACH OF CHILDREN
PARACETAMOL SUGAR-FREE
SUSPENSION 120mg in 5ml
Take ONE or TWO 5ml spoonfuls
every FOUR to SIX hours when
required for pain relief
SHAKE THE BOTTLE NOT MORE THAN
4 DOSES IN 24HRS Do not take
with any other PARACETAMOL
SIMON YOUNG 1/2
R SY W4A 11MAY15 AB53 100ml

PHARMACY DEPARTMENT
WHITCHURCH HOSPITAL
CHK
DISP

KEEP OUT OF THE REACH OF CHILDREN
products. Immediate medical
advice should be sought in the
case of an overdose, even if
the child seems well, because
of the risk of delayed,
serious liver damage.

SIMON YOUNG 2/2
R SY W4A 11MAY15 AB53 100ml

PHARMACY DEPARTMENT
WHITCHURCH HOSPITAL
CHK
DISP

*Medicines Management for Nurses at a Glance*. First Edition. Simon Young and Ben Pitcher. © 2016 John Wiley & Sons, Ltd. Published 2016 by John Wiley & Sons, Ltd.
www.ataglanceseries.com/nursing/medicinesmanagement

In common with managing medicines for elderly people (Chapter 45), there are special considerations to be made when managing medicines for children (Figure 44.1). Children can differ significantly from adults in many ways regarding approaches to managing medication. From a physiological and pharmacological perspective, children are not simply smaller versions of adults. Comprehension of information about medicines varies significantly; availability of dosage forms and a lack of licensed medicines for children present specific challenges.

## Key medicines management issues for children

### Dosing in children

The calculation of children's dosages are usually based on their age, body weight or in some cases their body surface area. With regard to age, the British National Formulary (BNF) and the British National Formulary for Children (BNFC) stratifies children into four distinct groups:

- Neonate (up to 1 month).
- Infant (up to 1 year).
- 1–6 years of age.
- 6–12 years of age.

#### *The perceptions of the child and their carer*

In addition to considering the needs of the child and the treatment of their medical condition, it is important to consider the person(s) who are responsible for that child's care. To overcome barriers to adherence, carers and children need clear explanations of the rationale behind a therapy. This may include an understanding of a drug's benefits, risks and side effects. A dosage regime that is clear and an understanding of the medicines management issues surrounding the use of the medicines (e.g. blood tests, follow-up monitoring, obtaining repeat medication) are also important.

As children mature, other factors may influence adherence, such as transitions to adulthood and peer pressure. Managing medicines in schools can be a complex matter but the Department of Health gives some guidance through 'Supporting Pupils at School with Medical Conditions' (https://www.gov.uk/government/uploads/system/uploads/attachment_data/file/349435/Statutory_guidance_on_supporting_pupils_at_school_with_medical_conditions.pdf, last accessed 6 August, 2015).

A child should be offered a formulation of medication that is suitable for their needs (e.g. in a form that they can easily swallow, has a 'pleasant' taste and takes into consideration their cultural needs). Disguising medicines is possible in some circumstances and some medicines may need to be mixed with foods. However, the full dose of the disguised medication might not be taken; also this practice can put a child off taking their medication and alter their perception of particular foodstuffs.

#### *Children's pharmacokinetics*

As children mature, their pharmacokinetic parameters (absorption, distribution, metabolism and excretion [ADME]) mature with them. The absorption of oral medicines is influenced by many factors such as gastric motility and gastro-intestinal pH. The gastric pH of children only reaches the same level as that of adults when they reach 2–3 years of age. Children's gastric emptying reaches the same level as that of adults at about 6 months. Despite this fact, children seem to respond to most oral medications as predicted. Intramuscular absorption in children and infants is faster than in neonates; factors such as blood flow to muscle influence the rate of drug absorption. The extent of absorption of medicines via the skin (transdermal route) is related to the thickness of the stratum corneum; this is thinner in children than in adults, allowing greater absorption. This may lead to a higher plasma level of drug, and an increased frequency and intensity of side effects than expected with adults.

Factors that influence drug distribution change with age. Total body water and extracellular fluid volume decrease (as a percentage of total body weight) as a child matures into adulthood. These in turn influence the dosing of some drugs.

Some enzymatic pathways responsible for metabolising drugs are absent or have a less significant presence in children than adults. In time, as a young patient reaches older infancy or young childhood, there is an increase in metabolic rate that can exceed that in some enzyme systems of an adult. Some drugs dosed at this time of life may require a higher mg/kg dosing regimen in a child to compensate for the increased metabolic rate. Children's metabolic pathways are also different from those of adults, and the livers of neonates, infants and children have different pathways for the phase II metabolism of drugs like paracetamol.

At birth, the kidneys have a functional immaturity that limits the capacity for renal excretion to take place. This immaturity is notable during infancy when the glomerular filtration rate is less than that in adults; it is not until about 8–12 months of age that glomerular and tubular processing matures. After this period of life, renal function is more akin to that of older children and adults.

Each of these parameters alone can influence drug dosing but in combination they are important in calculating starting doses and titration regimes for children.

### Other considerations

Medication contains many exipients besides the active ingredient. Many medications are labelled as being sugar free and do not contain cariogenic sugars (Figure 44.2). **Adult medicines may not be sugar free**; appropriate advice should be given on dental hygiene if they are given to children. Other excipients such as alcohol (ethanol) need to be carefully considered when used in children. Preservatives, colours and simple products such as lactose are present in medicines and may not be tolerated by certain patients (e.g. those with intolerances or allergies).

Despite some steps taken to improve the situation, there are few medicines specifically licensed for children. Most medicines used in children are practice adaptations with a limited evidence base.

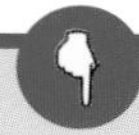

#### Clinical pointers

Relevant National Service Frameworks (NSFs) exist for children. If your role involves work with children, try reading the NSFs and considering their recommendations and markers of good practice with regard to managing medicines.

# Medicines management in elderly people

**Figure 45.1** Some considerations for using medications in older patients

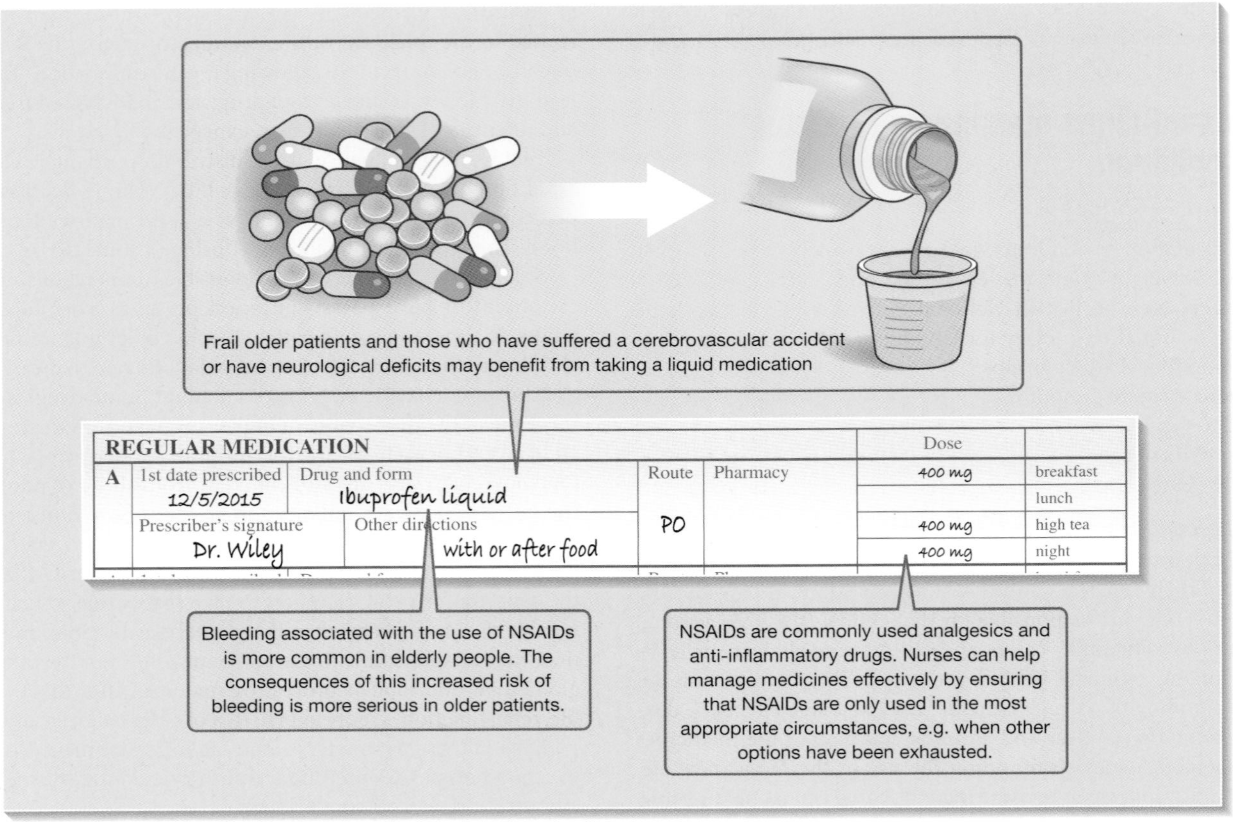

Frail older patients and those who have suffered a cerebrovascular accident or have neurological deficits may benefit from taking a liquid medication

| REGULAR MEDICATION | | | | | Dose | |
|---|---|---|---|---|---|---|
| A | 1st date prescribed<br>12/5/2015 | Drug and form<br>Ibuprofen liquid | Route | Pharmacy | 400 mg | breakfast |
| | | | | | | lunch |
| | Prescriber's signature<br>Dr. Wiley | Other directions<br>with or after food | PO | | 400 mg | high tea |
| | | | | | 400 mg | night |

Bleeding associated with the use of NSAIDs is more common in elderly people. The consequences of this increased risk of bleeding is more serious in older patients.

NSAIDs are commonly used analgesics and anti-inflammatory drugs. Nurses can help manage medicines effectively by ensuring that NSAIDs are only used in the most appropriate circumstances, e.g. when other options have been exhausted.

It is estimated that there are more than 10 million people in the UK who are over 65 years of age. Recent projections demonstrate that the number will increase by 5.5 million by 2030 and by 19 million by 2050. This has far-reaching implications for society as a whole and especially for health care.

In safely managing medicines, many considerations need to made from a nursing perspective. One important consideration is that of age. In caring for patients, the healthcare professional must take the necessary steps to ensure that the way in which medicines are used and managed is appropriate for each **individual** patient (Figure 45.1). However, when managing medicines for older patients, there are some key factors to consider that should influence a nurse's actions.

## National Service Frameworks

A 'National Service Framework (NSF) for Older People' was published in 2001. The framework has a broad scope exploring appropriate contexts of care for older patients but it explicitly mentions medicines management as a fundamental component of each of the NSF standards. More detail is provided about medicines use in an associated booklet called 'Medicines and Older People'. This document explores particular issues for medicines management for older patients, some of which are within the direct influence of healthcare professionals. Others are directed at issues such as ensuring older patients are fairly represented in clinical trials in order that the potential risks and benefits of using medicines in older patients are fully understood. Not considering the needs of patients in this context may contribute to an indirect form of ageism.

## Key medicines management issues for elderly patients

### Polypharmacy and multiple chronic illnesses

Elderly patients are statistically more likely to have chronic medical conditions (and often multiple chronic conditions); this, in turn, can lead to the requirement to take many medications. Increasing the number of medications taken increases the risk of adverse drug reactions (ADRs); e.g. side effects and drug interactions. Medications for older patients should be reviewed regularly to ensure that the target benefits derived from their use are being attained and the risks minimised. In addition, it is important that the reviews consider medicines that are **omitted** from a patient's medication list. Suboptimal treatment of conditions such as hypercholesterolemia can lead to longer-term problems that are costly to the individual patient. Typically, some groups of medicines such as antidepressants and antithrombotic treatments are under-used in older patients.

There is a shift in emphasis to using preventative medication strategies in modern Western health care (e.g. using antihypertensive agents to reduce the risk of more serious cardiovascular disease). Reviewing the appropriateness of these medications is extremely important. Particular care should be taken to ensure that patients who have poor prognoses or are in poor states of health are not taking medication from which they will see no benefit.

## Ageing

Elderly patients can demonstrate some considerable changes in pharmacokinetic parameters when compared with younger adults. These can result in a significant difference in response to drugs. This is one of the reasons why starting doses are lower in elderly people and dose titrations are often undertaken in a more considered fashion. Ageing can influence many aspects of ADME (absorption, distribution, metabolism and excretion) but excretion is the most greatly affected in the older patient. A decline in renal function is a manifestation of age: older patients typically excrete drugs more slowly. Factors such as dehydration, acute decline in renal function associated with illness, drugs with narrow therapeutic indices and those that are almost entirely renally excreted must be used with more caution in older patents. The British National Formulary (BNF) outlines clearly the consideration to be made for each drug agent. In addition, some drugs need to be monitored more carefully for signs of hepatic impairment. There is limited information available on the importance of pharmacodynamic changes that occur with age.

Other physical manifestations (e.g. muscle weakness) may be related to the natural ageing process and not a disease process that needs treatment with medication. Older patients exhibit greater sensitivity to some groups of drugs (e.g. benzodiazepines). Elderly patients are also more vulnerable to specific ADRs (e.g. to non-steroidal anti-inflammatory drugs [NSAIDs]), as bleeding is more common (and typically more serious) within this age group. The influence of NSAIDs on renal function can also adversely influence cardiovascular parameters.

## Adherence

Adherence to agreed medication regimes can be challenging for all patients. It is estimated that between a third and a half of all medicines prescribed for long-term illness are not taken as recommended.

Memory problems in older patients may be an important barrier to adhering to a medication regime. Patients with swallowing difficulties may have problems with swallowing some forms of medicine. Options exist if patients have swallowing difficulties, but these must also be carefully reviewed. Soluble or dispersible tablets and sachets may be used, but they may have higher sodium content and therefore not be appropriate for all patients. Liquid medicines are also used, but not all medicines are available as liquids and the bespoke manufacture of liquid medicines ('specials') can be costly. Crushing medicines is an option; however, the manufacturers of most medicines cannot typically advocate such an approach. Crushing medication can influence the desired outcome and produce dust that can affect the administering nurse.

Older patients with hearing or visual impairment may have difficulty listening to or reading instructions. Difficulty accessing a pharmacy or surgery and complex repeat prescribing systems can be barriers to obtaining medication. Similarly, conditions such as arthritis and other joint disease may be significant barriers to adherence if child proof lid or small tablets are used.

# Medicines management in people with hepatic and renal impairment

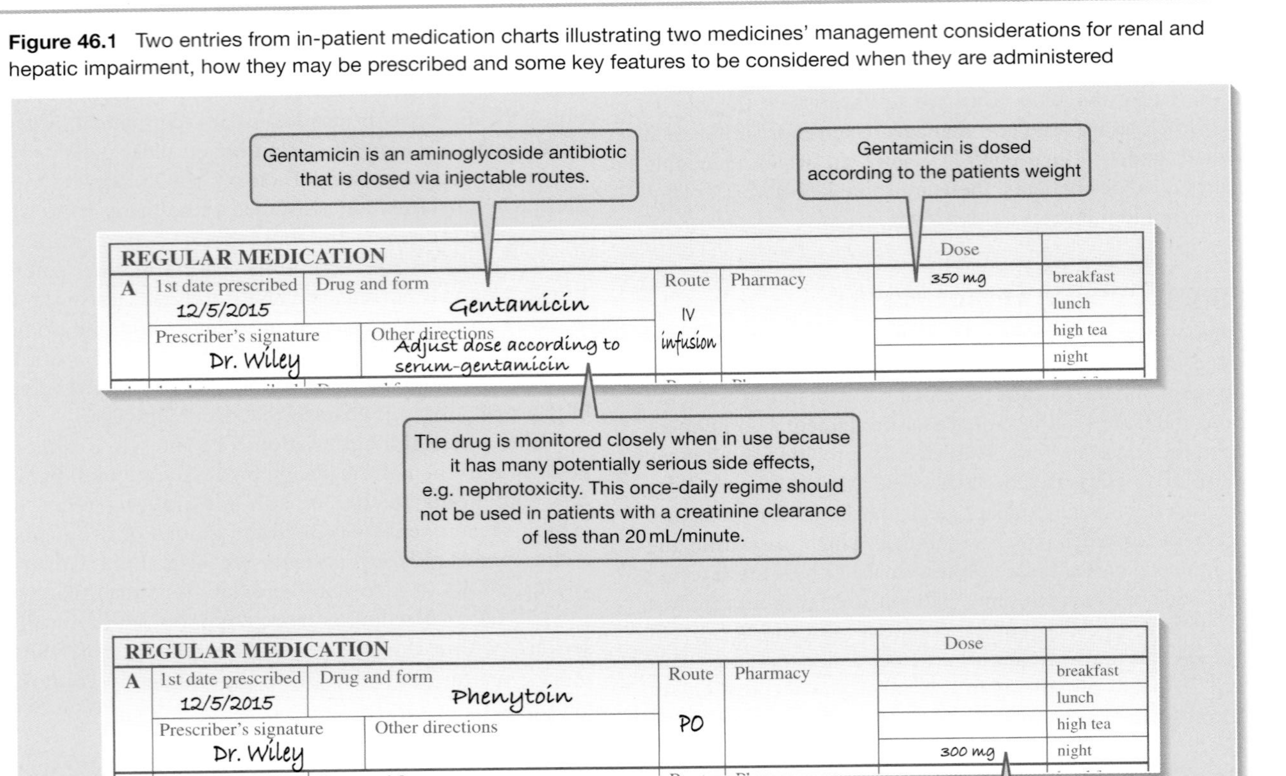


**Figure 46.1** Two entries from in-patient medication charts illustrating two medicines' management considerations for renal and hepatic impairment, how they may be prescribed and some key features to be considered when they are administered

In order for the body to deal with medication, from a pharmacokinetic perspective, both hepatic and renal function are important elements in medicines management. The liver is the organ that is primarily responsible for the metabolism of drugs and the kidneys for the excretion of drugs. Most drugs will undergo various degrees of hepatic and renal processing. When managing medicines, degrees of hepatic and renal impairment influence dosing and medicines selection (Figure 46.1).

If there is a loss of hepatic or renal function, pharmacological knowledge is important. At least two questions need to be asked about the choice of a medication. For example, in renal or hepatic impairment:

1 Does the drug need to excreted by the kidney or metabolised by the liver, and to what extent do adjustments need to be made if that is the case?
2 Is the drug renally toxic or hepatotoxic? If so, can another drug or member of the drug family be used to avoid the toxic effects?

Lack of adjustment will probably lead to an increased risk of side effects and potentially more organ damage if the drug is hepatotoxic or nephrotoxic.

In addition to the two features already mentioned, other specific considerations need to be made. If kidney or hepatic function is severely compromised, then drug use should be kept to an absolute minimum.

## Managing medicines in hepatic impairment

The liver has many functions and drug metabolism is only one. The liver has a reasonable reserve and hepatic function has to be severely compromised before drug metabolic function declines to a clinically significant level. Liver function tests are not an accurate guide to the degree to which an individual's metabolism of an individual drug is being influenced. In severe liver disease, hypoalbuminurea can be detected. This can be important when considering what influence albumin has on the availability of highly protein-bound agents such as phenytoin. Lower blood albumin will lead to more free (unbound) drug in the bloodstream and expose the patient to an increased risk of toxicity.

The liver is responsible for the production of key clotting factors. Any hepatic compromise that leads to a change in clotting factor production will alter sensitivity to anticoagulant medication such as warfarin.

## Managing medicines in renal impairment

Reduced renal function can have a significant impact on managing medicines. If renal function is compromised, then the patient's capacity to excrete drugs is usually decreased. Often, some adjustment has to be made if the drug or its active metabolites are renally excreted. Failure to make the correct adjustment will increase the likelihood of side effects and toxicity associated with the drug.

There are many causes for decline in renal function but the most common to be considered is that of age. Renal function tends to decline with age, and a patient may have some level of renal failure even if the markers of renal function are within the normal physiological ranges. In renal impairment, dose adjustment should be made in both individual doses and loading doses of affected drugs.

## Examples of when drug and renal function are considered

### Digoxin

Digoxin is the most widely used drug from the cardiac glycoside family. The drug is used to treat arrhythmias such as atrial fibrillation and heart failure. Digoxin distribution (and elimination) are changed in patients with renal impairment. The drug is primarily eliminated by renal excretion; 60–80% of the drug is excreted unchanged in urine. The British National Formulary (BNF) and summary of product characteristics (SPC) suggest that the dose should be reduced in renal impairment and that therapeutic drug monitoring may need to be undertaken to maintain a safe and effective drug plasma concentration. The drug's toxicity is further increased by electrolyte disturbances, which may be influenced by renal impairment and the presence of other drugs concomitantly administered (e.g. diuretics).

### Gentamicin

Gentamicin has a narrow therapeutic index. There are two serious side effects associated with gentamicin use: dose-related ototoxicity (deafness) and nephrotoxicity. The drug is eliminated unchanged via renal excretion so monitoring renal function is vital to managing the therapy effectively. The fact that the drug is nephrotoxic also has a bearing because this may adversely influence ongoing therapy.

### Lithium

Lithium is termed a mood-stabilising agent. The drug is used to treat mood disorders such as bipolar disorder and mental health disorders with mania and depression. It is another drug with a narrow therapeutic index whose effectiveness and safety are measured by therapeutic drug monitoring. Because lithium is a simple cation (positively charged ion), it is entirely eliminated by excretion and undergoes no metabolic transformation. Dehydration, changes in renal function, drug therapy (such as diuretics, non-steroidal anti-inflammatory drugs [NSAIDs] and angiotensin converting enzyme [ACE] inhibitors) can all interfere with the body's clearance of lithium.

One of the requirements of lithium therapy is that renal function is monitored every 6 months (more frequently with renal impairment). This is part of the National Patient Safety Agency's guidance, 'Safer Lithium Therapy' (http://www.nrls.npsa.nhs.uk/alerts/?entryid45=65426, last accessed 6 August, 2015).

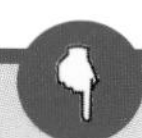

**Clinical pointers**

The BNF and the SPC have clear guidelines that point to drugs that may cause problems for patients with hepatic or renal disease. The BNF gives a detailed explanation of how creatinine clearance and estimated glomerular filtration rate are used in adjusting drug dose.

# Drug interactions

**Figure 47.1** An entry from an in-patient medication chart illustrating an interaction between two drugs. The excretion of lithium is adversely affected by the NSAID naproxen and the two drugs are usually not co-administered

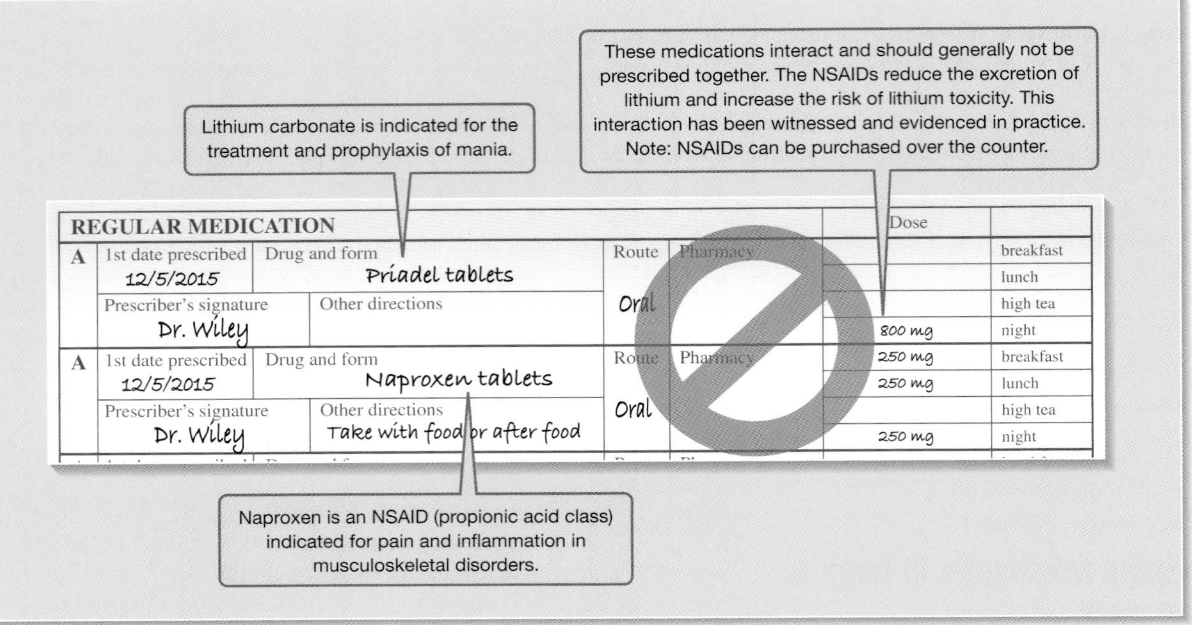


**Figure 47.2** Types of drug interactions

| Type of interaction | Examples from practice |
|---|---|
| **Drug – drug** | NSAIDs vs. lithium<br>Carbamazepine vs. combined oral contraceptives |
| **Drug – food** | Warfarin vs. leafy green vegetables<br>Simvastatin vs. grapefruit juice |
| **Drug – smoking** | Clozapine vs. smoking<br>Theophylline vs. smoking |
| **Drug – alcohol** | Disulfiram vs. ethanol<br>Metronidazole vs. ethanol |

A **drug interaction** is a situation in which a substance (often, but not exclusively, another drug) influences the activity of a drug when both are administered concomitantly (Figure 47.1). The effects of the drug can be increased, decreased or may produce a new effect that neither drug produces on its own. Drug interactions occur inside the human body in contrast to drug incompatibilities, which occur inside fluid containers or infusion lines and are often visible to the naked eye. Drug incompatibilities occur when chemical components of the drug or excipients react with each other before or during administration. This can occur at the preparation stage or when multiple drugs are administered via the same point of access.

## Why are drug interactions important?

Drug interactions are a subset of adverse drug reactions (ADRs; Chapter 48). They are an important cause of avoidable iatrogenic disease. Patients who take many drugs (polypharmacy) are at greater risk of interactions than those who take fewer medications. Predicting when drug interactions are clinically relevant is particularly difficult and requires a degree of understanding of pharmacology, physiology and pathophysiological processes.

The British National Formulary (BNF) provides a list of known drug interactions in it's Appendix 1. However, there are many drug interactions that are as yet unrecognised. The absence of the documentation of an interaction in texts like the BNF does not automatically mean that a given drug combination is safe. Recognising drug interactions is challenging and often requires the support of an experienced colleague such as a pharmacist or a specialist who has dealt with interactions in that field of practice.

## Classification of drug interactions

The BNF classifies drug interactions as either pharmacodynamic or pharmacokinetic in nature. Pharmacodynamic interactions occur with drugs that share a similar mechanism of action. An example of this is the interaction between $beta_2$ agonists (e.g. salbutamol) that stimulate beta-receptors, and beta-blockers (e.g. propranolol) that block beta-receptors. The 'blocking' effect of the propranolol prevents the salbutamol gaining access to beta-receptors. If this influence is felt in the airways, then the salbutamol will be unable to exert its bronchodilator effect.

Pharmacokinetic drug interactions occur when one drug alters the pharmacokinetic parameters of another drug. The interacting drug influences or affects the absorption, distribution, metabolism or excretion (ADME) of another drug. For example, components of antacids (usually $Mg^{2+}$ or $Ca^{2+}$), when co-administered with tetracycline, binds to tetracycline and reduces its absorption.

Many drugs can influence the capacity of the liver to metabolise other agents. Drugs such as carbamazepine, rifampicin and sodium valproate have this effect and consequently have a list of interactions associated with their use. Other clinically important interactions occur when a drug influences the metabolism and excretion of other drugs. Diuretics can alter the rates of renal excretion of other drugs. Lithium is primarily renally excreted and any drug (e.g. non-steroidal anti-inflammatory drugs [NSAIDs]) that influences the rate and extent of lithium excretion can lead to lithium toxicity.

Figure 47.2 illustrates that it is not only drugs that interact with each other: non-drug substances can influence outcomes of drug therapy. The BNF uses the black dot (•) symbol to classify interactions that are 'potentially serious and where concomitant administration of the drugs involved should be avoided (or only undertaken with caution and appropriate monitoring)' and the BNF online uses red text to indicate these serious interactions. Many texts refer to the severity of drug interactions and try to distinguish between theoretical interactions and those that occur more frequently in practice. Some drug interactions can lead to fatal consequences, such as the interaction between certain monoamine-oxidase inhibitors (MAOIs) and the tricyclic antidepressants. By contrast, some drug interactions are beneficial, such as the co-administration of benserazide with levodopa to maximise the effectiveness of the levodopa.

## Underlying factors

There appear to be certain underlying factors that influence a patient's susceptibility to drug interactions. There are person-dependent factors and drug-dependent factors. Older people, children and the critically unwell seem to be more susceptible to drug interactions. Factors such as altered pharmacokinetics, multiple chronic diseases and complex polypharmacy may play a role. Certain drugs, such as lithium and digoxin, have a narrow therapeutic index and, as such, small changes in their metabolism or excretion can result in negative outcomes. Other drugs with less 'conventional' pharmacokinetic profiles, such as phenytion, are more commonly involved in drug interactions.

### Clinical pointers

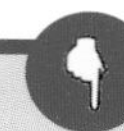

If one drug increases the effectiveness of another, then you may observe an increase in the intensity of side effects associated with that drug. This highlights the importance of knowing the side effects of the drugs you administer. You may be in a position to spot potentially serious interactions and intervene in a timely fashion before the situation deteriorates.

Some medications interact with smoking. This is important because, when opportunities present, patients are encouraged to give up smoking for the wider health benefits. Stopping or starting smoking may influence drug therapy and can be considered part of managing medicines safely. Typically, it is the carcinogenic 'tar' components that interact with medication (via an interference with hepatic metabolic processes), not the nicotine. Patients who are using nicotine replacement therapy may still be susceptible to changes in drug effectiveness.

# Adverse drug reactions

**Figure 48.1** An entry from an in-patient medication chart illustrating the prescribing of the antipsychotic medication clozapine and the co-prescribing of three other drugs that are used to manage the side effects of clozapine


This medication is used to manage the constipation associated with clozapine's use
This medication is used to manage the hypersalivation associated with clozapine's use.
This medication is used to manage the tachycardia associated with clozapine's use.


| REGULAR MEDICATION | | | | | | Dose | |
|---|---|---|---|---|---|---|---|
| A | 1st date prescribed 12/5/2015 | Drug and form Clozapine | | Route Oral | Pharmacy | | breakfast |
| | | | | | | | lunch |
| | Prescriber's signature Dr. Wiley | Other directions | | | | | high tea |
| | | | | | | 400 mg | night |
| A | 1st date prescribed 12/5/2015 | Drug and form Senna tablets | | Route | Pharmacy | ii | breakfast |
| | | | | | | | lunch |
| | Prescriber's signature Dr. Wiley | Other directions | | | | | high tea |
| | | | | | | ii | night |
| A | 1st date prescribed 12/5/2015 | Drug and form Hyoscine hydrobromide tablets | | Route | Pharmacy | 300 micrograms | breakfast |
| | | | | | | 300 micrograms | lunch |
| | Prescriber's signature Dr. Wiley | Other directions | | | | | high tea |
| | | | | | | 300 micrograms | night |
| A | 1st date prescribed 12/5/2015 | Drug and form Atenolol tablets | | Route | Pharmacy | 50 mg | breakfast |
| | | | | | | | lunch |
| | Prescriber's signature Dr. Wiley | Other directions | | | | | high tea |
| | | | | | | | night |

An adverse drug reaction (ADR) is an unwanted or harmful reaction that occurs after administration of a drug and is **suspected** or known to be due to the drug. These may cause harm or discomfort and may require additional medications to be prescribed to manage the unwanted effects (Figure 48.1). Aronson and Edwards extend the definition to:

> *an appreciably harmful or unpleasant reaction, resulting from an intervention related to the use of a medicinal product, which predicts hazard from future administration and warrants prevention or specific treatment, or alteration of the dosage regimen, or withdrawal of the product.*
>
> (Source: Edwards, I.R. and Aronson, J.K., 2000. Adverse drug reactions: definitions, diagnosis, and management, Lancet, October 7, 356(9237): 1255–9. http://www.sciencedirect.com/science/article/pii/S0140673600027999, last accessed 6 August, 2015)

None of these definitions point to the important aspect of harm that is intentional overdose; these definitions look at adverse reactions when drugs are used at therapeutic doses in humans.

## Why are adverse drug reactions important?

Research and audit work have clearly demonstrated that ADRs are an important cause of morbidity (ill health) and mortality (death) in medicine. When exploring the nature of iatrogenic disease, medicines are often the root cause. Spotting adverse drug reactions is important but not always an easy task; the vigilance of the nurse is important. The nurse should be especially familiar with the ADRs of drugs in their particular therapeutic area.

## Classification of adverse drug reactions

In order to better understand ADRs and how to manage them, a classification system is used. Typically, ADRs are classified as either Type A or Type B adverse reactions. Edwards and Aronson (2000) extend this to Types A–F:

Type A
(Augmented) reactions are normal pharmacological effects that are undesirable.

Type B
(Bizarre) reactions are effects unrelated to the known pharmacology of the drug.

Type C
(Chronic) reactions are dose related and time related.

Type D
(Delayed) reactions that occur sometime after stopping treatment.

Type E
(End of use) reactions related to abrupt drug withdrawal.

Type F
(Failure of therapy).

In the UK, we use the Type A and B classifications in relation to pharmacovigilance (the branch of pharmacology focused on detecting, assessing, understanding and preventing long- and short-term adverse effects of medicines).

## The features of Type A reactions

Type A ADRs are usually dose dependent (typically, the higher the dose, the more pronounced the adverse effect), fairly predictable (and related to the known pharmacology of the medicine) and an important cause of morbidity. The incidence of Type A ADRs is relatively high in comparison to Type B ADRs. Type A ADRs will usually respond to the reduction of a medicine dose or the stopping of a medicine if the reaction is severe.

Salbutamol, when used to treat asthma, acts as a bronchodilator (see Chapter 21). In addition to this desirable effect, it also causes tachycardia and tremor, both of which are Type A ADRs that relate to the pharmacology of β agonists. These side effects become more prominent where the dose used is high (e.g. when the medicine is nebulised) and subsides as the medicine leaves the body.

## The features of Type B reactions

Type B (bizarre) ADRs are usually relatively rare occurrences. They are difficult to predict because they are idiosyncratic and the reactions do not usually relate to the pharmacology of the medicine. The reactions are not dose dependent and relatively small doses can trigger the ADR. The reactions witnessed in Type B ADRs are often severe responses and can quickly become fatal if not spotted and the symptoms managed. Fortunately, their incidence in practice is low in comparison to Type A ADRs. Examples seen in practice include penicillin allergy.

Because Type B ADRs are rare, they are not always detected in the initial phases of drug testing and are often only encountered when the drug goes to market. This is one reason why the process of pharmacovigilance in so important in drug safety. It puts a responsibility on healthcare professionals to be aware that signs and symptoms in a patient may be a 'new' emerging ADR that is previously undocumented.

## Predisposing factors

Certain groups of patients are more vulnerable to ADRs than others and certain factors can influence the likelihood that a patient will suffer ADRs. An obvious factor to consider is multiple drug therapy (polypharmacy). Patients who take a list of medications are more likely to suffer side effects associated with one drug that may in turn influence another (a drug interaction). Diuretics that cause the loss of sodium ions ($Na^+$) and potassium ions ($K^+$) can influence the efficacy of medications like digoxin whose mechanisms of action are dependent on the presence of the correct concentration of certain ions.

In general, older patients are more vulnerable to ADRs than younger adults. This is partly because the factors that influence pharmacokinetics (absorption, distribution, metabolism and excretion [ADME]) and pharmacodynamics in older patients differ from those in younger adults.

Genetic and/or racial differences and the development of intercurrent disease may also be influencing factors in the development of ADRs.

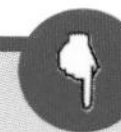

### Clinical pointers

The black triangle symbol (▼) identifies newly licensed medicines or medicines that are undergoing more intensive monitoring by the Medicines and Healthcare products Regulatory Agency (MHRA). The black triangle symbol appears in the British National Formulary (BNF), summary of product characteristics (SPC), patient information leaflet (PIL) and on all promotional literature for relevant medicines, with a brief explanation of what it means. Pay particular attention to these medicines – our knowledge of their ADRs is limited (or we have concerns over their safety) in comparison to those that do not have the (▼) identifier.

# Pharmacovigilance

**Figure 49.1** 'Yellow Card' notification for suspected adverse drug reactions. *Source: Yellow Card reporting form. © Crown copyright. Reproduced under OGL 3.0.*

It is important to note the use of the word 'suspected'. You do not need to be certain of the nature of the ADR or if the drug is definitely to blame.

A Yellow Card reporting form produced by the MHRA. This is a standard form used by healthcare professionals to report ADRs. There is also a version that is available for members of the public to use.

In Confidence

**YellowCard**
COMMISSION ON HUMAN MEDICINES (CHM)

It's easy to report online at
www.mhra.gov.uk/yellowcard

MHRA

**REPORT OF SUSPECTED ADVERSE DRUG REACTIONS**

If you suspect an adverse reaction may be related to one or more drugs/vaccines/complementary remedies, please complete this Yellow Card. See 'Adverse reactions to drugs' section in the British National Formulary (BNF) or **www.mhra.gov.uk/yellowcard** for guidance. Do not be put off reporting because some details are not known.

**PATIENT DETAILS** Patient Initials:________ Sex: M / F Is the patient pregnant? Y / N Ethnicity:________

Age (at time of reaction):______ Weight (kg):______ Identification number (e.g. Practice or Hospital Ref):________

**SUSPECTED DRUG(S)/VACCINE(S)**

| Drug/Vaccine (Brand if known) | Batch | Route | Dosage | Date started | Date stopped | Prescribed for |
|---|---|---|---|---|---|---|
| | | | | | | |
| | | | | | | |

**SUSPECTED REACTION(S)** Please describe the reaction(s) and any treatment given. (Please attach additional pages if necessary):

**Outcome**
Recovered
Recovering
Continuing
Other

Date reaction(s) started:________ Date reaction(s) stopped:________
Do you consider the reactions to be serious? Yes / No
If yes, please indicate why the reaction is considered to be serious (please tick all that apply):
- Patient died due to reaction
- Life threatening
- Congenital abnormality
- Involved or prolonged inpatient hospitalisation
- Involved persistent or significant disability or incapacity
- Medically significant; please give details:________

If the reactions were not serious according to the categories above, how bad was the suspected reaction?
- Mild
- Unpleasant, but did not affect everyday activities
- Bad enough to affect everyday activities

**OTHER DRUG(S) (including self-medication and complementary remedies)**
Did the patient take any other medicines/vaccines/complementary remedies in the last 3 months prior to the reaction? Yes / No
If yes, please give the following information if known:

| Drug/Vaccine (Brand if known) | Batch | Route | Dosage | Date started | Date stopped | Prescribed for |
|---|---|---|---|---|---|---|
| | | | | | | |
| | | | | | | |
| | | | | | | |
| | | | | | | |
| | | | | | | |

**Additional relevant information** e.g. medical history, test results, known allergies, rechallenge (if performed). For reactions relating to use of a medicine during pregnancy please state all other drugs taken during pregnancy, the last menstrual period, information on previous pregnancies, ultrasound scans, any delivery complications, birth defects or developmental concerns.

Please list any medicines obtained from the internet:

**REPORTER DETAILS**
Name and Professional Address:________
Postcode:________ Tel No:________
Email:________
Speciality:________
Signature:________ Date:________

**CLINICIAN (if not the reporter)**
Name and Professional Address:________
Postcode:________ Tel No:________
Email:________
Speciality:________
Signature:________ Date:________

Information on adverse drug reactions received by the MHRA can be downloaded at **www.mhra.gov.uk/daps**
Stay up-to-date on the latest advice for the safe use of medicines with our monthly bulletin *Drug Safety Update* at **www.mhra.gov.uk/drugsafetyupdate**

Please attach additional pages if necessary. Send to: FREEPOST YELLOW CARD (no other address details required)

## What is pharmacovigilance? Why is it important?

'Pharmacovigilance' is the term applied to the scientific study of monitoring drug safety. Drug safety is an important consideration before a drug is licensed and marketed. Clinical trials and related studies are important in establishing baseline safety issues and making preliminary risk–benefit analyses for using drugs. In addition, there is a process that considers the collection, detection and monitoring of adverse events for pharmaceutical products while they are on the market. The process is a scientific exploration of drug efficacy and safety when it is used in the wider patient population.

Before marketing, only some of a drug's adverse drug reactions (ADRs) will have been established. Some only emerge when a drug is used in a more diverse population of humans. However, pharmacovigilance is not only about spotting new ADRs: some drugs may cause ADRs of greater severity or frequency in certain patient groups. The Medicines and Healthcare Products Regulatory Agency (MHRA) gathers data on the ADRs of all drugs used in the UK. If a problematic pattern of side effects emerges, the MHRA can determine what action, if any, is needed in order that the drug can safely continue to be used, and hence optimise the drug's efficacy and minimise risk. The MHRA also informs healthcare professionals of their findings and any action needed.

## What methods are used to monitor the safety of medicines on the market?

A number of methods are used to continually monitor the safety of medicines. The increase in use of technology in medical and academic publishing means that sharing information about the safety of medicines can occur globally. Regulatory authorities and pharmaceutical companies worldwide are able to share pharmacovigilance information. Case reports, larger epidemiological studies, searches of the medical literature and healthcare databases allow relevant data to be mined regarding ADRs. One of the most important methods of gathering data is the spontaneous reporting scheme (such as the MHRA/Commission on Human Medicines [CHM] Yellow Card Scheme [Figure 49.1]).

Spontaneous ADR reporting is an important method for post-marketing surveillance of medicines. The schemes that operate worldwide provide important data for monitoring and (if necessary) modifying drug use. Essentially, anyone who suspects an ADR can report it through the Yellow Card Scheme and the MHRA/CHM can use that data to build a profile of a medicine's safety.

Patients, carers or parents can report any side effects they have experienced from a medicine. Healthcare professionals are expected to report **ALL** suspected ADRs for new medicines or those that are being monitored closely (black triangle [▼] drugs). For more established medicines, health professionals report only **serious** suspected adverse reactions. The level of seriousness of a reaction is defined by the Yellow Card Scheme but it includes increased duration of stay in hospital as well as death.

The information collected through the Yellow Card Scheme is an important tool in helping monitor safety. Yellow Card reports are evaluated, together with additional sources of information to detect previously unidentified hazards or side effects. If a new side effect is identified, information is carefully considered in the context of the overall side-effect profile for the medicine, and how it compares with other medicines used to treat the same condition (i.e. reports do not automatically require punitive responses).

## Possible actions to be taken

The MHRA can undertake a number of actions to change the way a medicine is used, in response to safety concerns:

1 Change the way a medicine is perceived/used

The MHRA/CHM can, in response to data, take the following actions:

- Make changes to warnings in product information or on a package label.
- Restrict the indications for use of a medicine.
- Change the legal status of a medicine (e.g. from over the counter to prescription only).
- In rare circumstances, remove a medicine from the market, if its risks are found to outweigh its benefits.

The MHRA can enforce these actions; however, the pharmaceutical companies most frequently make appropriate changes to the use of their products if evidence supports that change. It is in the industry's best interest that medicines are used to their best effect.

2 Communicate with professionals and/or patients

The regulatory authorities can provide feedback by updating patient information leaflets (PILs) and summaries of product characteristics (SPCs), cascading safety updates to healthcare professionals and providing educational updates. This feedback mechanism ensures that healthcare professionals have the most current information on drug safety that will be reflected in changes to the British National Formulary (BNF). For this reason, practitioners should always use the most up-to-date version of the BNF or other relevant publications.

### Clinical pointers

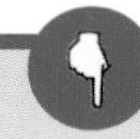

Pharmacovigilance is an important part of every healthcare professional's role and it is often the nurse who will spot emerging side effects as part of the work of providing care. Look at the MHRA's website and the BNF, and study the Yellow Card reporting scheme and the forms used to report ADRs. Many healthcare professionals are reluctant to fill in the forms. What would happen to drug safety if none of us cared about ADRs?

The MHRA has other roles. It also regulates medical devices, advanced therapy medicinal products and blood products, so its role in safely managing patients extends beyond medicines alone. It will produce other datasets and pieces of information that will have an impact on your practice as a nurse.

# Classification of medicines

Figure 50.1 A range of medications and their different strengths and dosages in different classifications

| Drug | GSL | | P-medicine* | | POM | |
|---|---|---|---|---|---|---|
| **Ibuprofen tablets** | Strength: | **200 mg** | Strength: | **400 mg** | Strength: | **600 mg** |
| | Dose: | **400 mg** | Dose: | **400 mg** | Dose: | **600 mg** |
| | Daily dose: | **up to 1200 mg** | Daily dose: | **up to 1200 mg** | Daily dose: | **up to 2400 mg** |
| | Amount supplied: | **16 tablets** | Amount supplied: | **48 tablets** | Amount supplied: | **determined by prescriber** |
| **Omeprazole capsules** | Not available | | Strength: | **10 mg** | Strength: | **40 mg** |
| | | | Dose: | **20 mg** | Dose: | **60 mg** |
| | | | Daily dose: | **20 mg** | Daily dose: | **60 mg** |
| | | | Amount supplied: | **28 tablets** | Amount supplied: | **determined by prescriber** |
| | | | Available since 2003 | | | |

* P-medicines have a restricted range of indications compared with the POM versions, e.g. Omeprazole (P) for relief of reflux-like symptoms such as heartburn in adults aged 18 years and over for a maximum period of 4 weeks.

The way medicines are used in health care is governed by several factors; these include professional standards (e.g. the Nursing and Midwifery Council (NMC) 'Standards for Medicines Management'), workplace considerations (protocols and policies) and the laws that govern medicines' use. The most important piece of legislation that dictates how healthcare professionals behave with medicines is the Human Medicines Regulations 2012 (HMR).

The HMR is an all-encompassing piece of legislation that deals with a range of issues with regard to medicines use. It lays out important definitions: for example, it defines a medicine or medicinal product, outlines a range of issues such as medicine manufacture and pharmacovigilance, and specifies who has the authority to write prescriptions, how medicines can be imported or exported and how medicines are classified in the UK (Figure 50.1).

## Classification of medicines in the UK

The HMR defines three classifications of medicines in the UK:

**Prescription-only medicines (POMs)** cannot be sold or supplied except when there is a prescription written that authorises that transaction. Prescribers in modern health care include doctors, dentists and various types of nurse and pharmacist prescribers. This is the highest level of control exercised over medicine use because there are regulations that dictate what constitutes a prescription, who is authorised to deal with the medicines that have been sold or supplied, how they are stored and what records must be kept with regard to those transactions. There are additional restrictions on the use of drugs that may be subject to misuse; these are known as 'controlled drugs' (CDs). Most drugs encountered in health care are POMs. A range of exceptions to the regulation exist to cover, for example, medication administration in emergencies, patient group directions (PGDs) and emergency supplies of medicines by pharmacists.

**General sales list medicines (GSLs)** are those with the lowest level of control over their sale and supply. They can be sold from any outlet that can be safely locked by the proprietor. The medicines can only be sold in their immediate and outer packing (i.e. individual strips or tablets should not be removed and sold separately). Medicines in this category will include paracetamol, cetirizine and ibuprofen. There are limitations set on the dosage, labelling, strength of product and pack sizes. These medicines are considered safe for patients to buy and use without professional healthcare advice.

**Pharmacy medicines (P-medicines)** can only be sold by a pharmacist or under the supervision of a pharmacist from a registered pharmacy premises. P-medicines are often lower-strength POMs intended for short-term use. Some GSLs may be available in larger pack sizes and sold as P-medicines. P-medicines usually have a fixed pack size and distinct packaging. Patients are able to select their own medications only with the advice (and approval) of a pharmacist. Examples include naproxen, co-codamol 8 mg/500 mg and omeprazole (proton pump inhibitor).

## Controlled drugs

The potential for the misuse of certain drugs gave rise to legislation that added levels of control to the use of these drugs. The Misuse of Drugs Act 1971 was designed to prevent the misuse of CDs by placing restriction on their possession, supply, manufacture, import and export. Groups of medicines included in the legislation encompass amphetamines, narcotic analgesics (e.g. diamorphine and morphine), benzodiazepines (e.g. diazepam; Chapter 24), anabolic steroids and growth hormones.

The Act sets CDs into four separate drug classes: Classes A–C and a temporary class. These classes define the level of penalties imposed for offences relating to these drugs and are intended to represent the harm the drug does. The temporary class gives the government and its advisers a means to categorise a drug in a timely fashion. This is important in the context of newer 'designer drugs' that do not fit into any of the other classes. Class A drugs, such as ecstasy, LSD and heroin, are subject to the harshest penalties and Class C agents, such as the benzodiazepines, the lowest.

In addition to the Misuse of Drugs Act 1971, the Misuse of Drugs Regulations 2001 govern the use of CDs in practice. Each CD is put into one of five schedules according to the level of control exercised over the drug or groups of drugs. Each category reflects the therapeutic utility of the drug involved and its potential for misuse:

Schedule 1 Houses drugs that currently have 'limited' medical uses (e.g. cannabis plant, coca leaf and LSD). In order to use a Schedule 1 CD in practice, a licence from the Home Office is required.

Schedule 2 Includes the opiates (e.g. morphine and pethidine). This schedule assigns particular requirements such as paperwork for acquisition of the drug, its safe storage, disposal and destruction, and relevant record keeping.

Schedule 3 Contains some synthetic opioids and other agents that are less liable to be misused and therefore do not require as strict a degree of control as those in Schedule 2. Typically, record keeping and storage and disposal have fewer restrictions than Schedule 2 agents.

Schedule 4 Applies mainly to certain benzodiazepines and anabolic steroids. Special considerations need to be made with regard to the safe destruction of some schedule 4 CDs.

Schedule 5 Includes drugs with lower 'strengths' of codeine and preparations containing dihydrocodeine. Some Schedule 5 CDs are available over the counter or for sale in pharmacies.

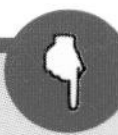

### Clinical pointers

Read the policies that centre on medicines management in relation to CDs. Some areas of practice place extra checks and balances to ensure safe CD use (e.g. involving two nurses in administration procedures and treating Schedule 4 CDs like those in Schedule 3).

# Index

Note: page numbers in *italics* refer to figures; those in **bold** to tables.




*Medicines Management for Nurses at a Glance.* First Edition. Simon Young and Ben Pitcher. © 2016 John Wiley & Sons, Ltd. Published 2016 by John Wiley & Sons, Ltd.
www.ataglanceseries.com/nursing/medicinesmanagement

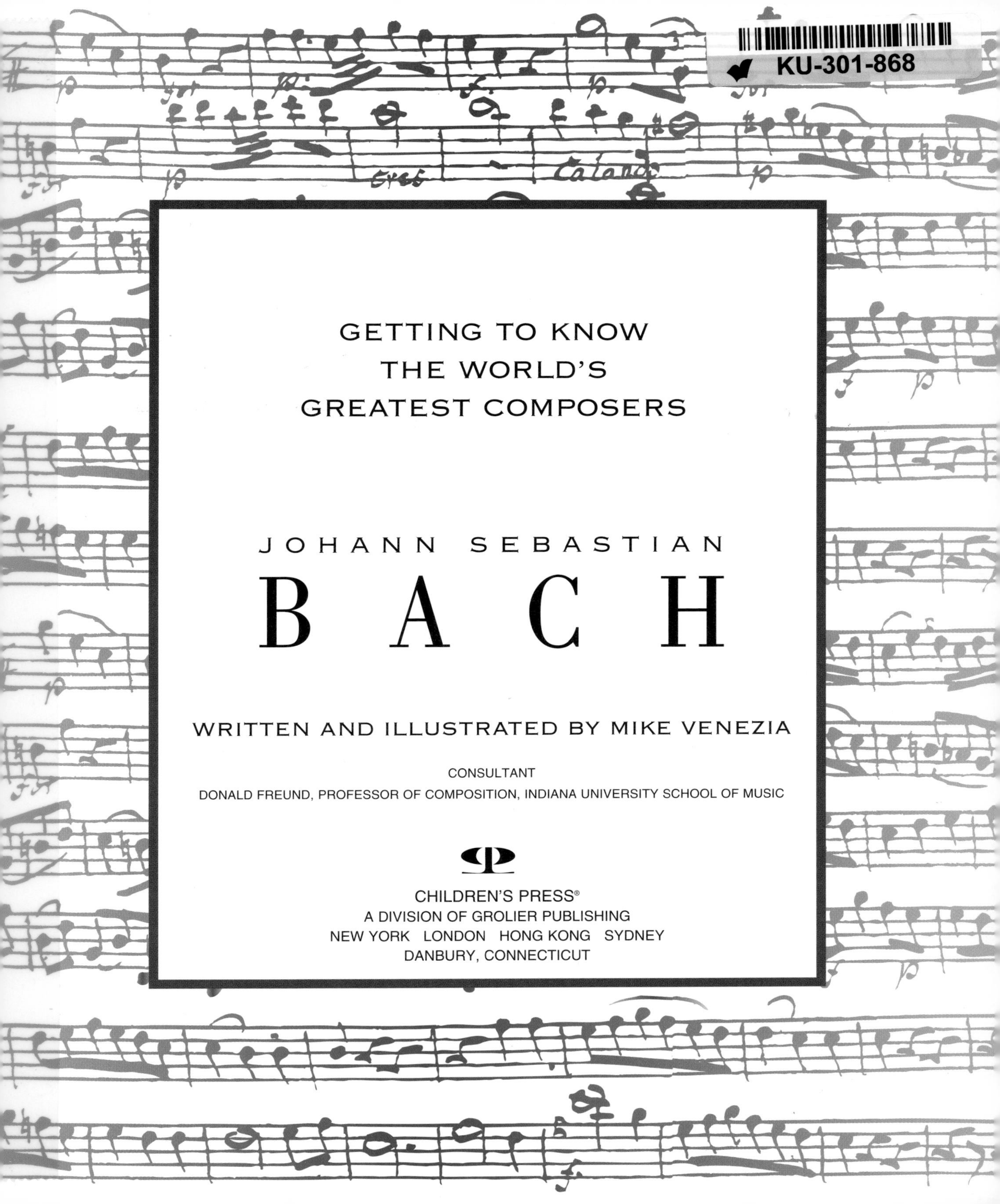


GETTING TO KNOW
THE WORLD'S
GREATEST COMPOSERS

# JOHANN SEBASTIAN BACH

WRITTEN AND ILLUSTRATED BY MIKE VENEZIA

CONSULTANT
DONALD FREUND, PROFESSOR OF COMPOSITION, INDIANA UNIVERSITY SCHOOL OF MUSIC

CHILDREN'S PRESS®
A DIVISION OF GROLIER PUBLISHING
NEW YORK LONDON HONG KONG SYDNEY
DANBURY, CONNECTICUT

*A special thanks to the Music Department at Grace Lutheran Church and School in River Forest, Illinois, especially Dr. Richard Hillert and Mr. John Folkening.*

Photographs ©: AKG London: 3, 18, 20, 24, 25, 27, 30, 31; bildarchiv preussischer kulturbesitz: 9; Corbis-Bettmann: 10, 14, 32; Erich Lessing/Art Resource, NY: 6 bottom; The Peirpont Morgan Library, Mary Flagler Cary Music Collection/Art Resource, NY: 21; Scala/Art Resource, NY: 6 top, 8.

Visit Children's Press on the Internet at:
http://publishing.grolier.com

Library of Congress Cataloging–in–Publication Data

Venezia, Mike.
Johann Sebastian Bach / written and illustrated by Mike Venezia.
p. cm. — (Getting to know the world's greatest composers)
ISBN 0-516-20760-1 (lib. bdg.) 0-516-26352-8 (pbk.)
1. Bach, Johann Sebastian, 1685-1750—Juvenile literature.
2. Composers—Germany—Biography—Juvenile literature. I. Title.
II. Series: Venezia, Mike. Getting to know the world's greatest composers.
ML3930.B2V46 1998
780' .92—dc21
[B}

97-25756
CIP
AC MN


Printed in the United States of America.
2 3 4 5 6 7 8 9 0 R 07 06 05 04 03 02 01 00 99

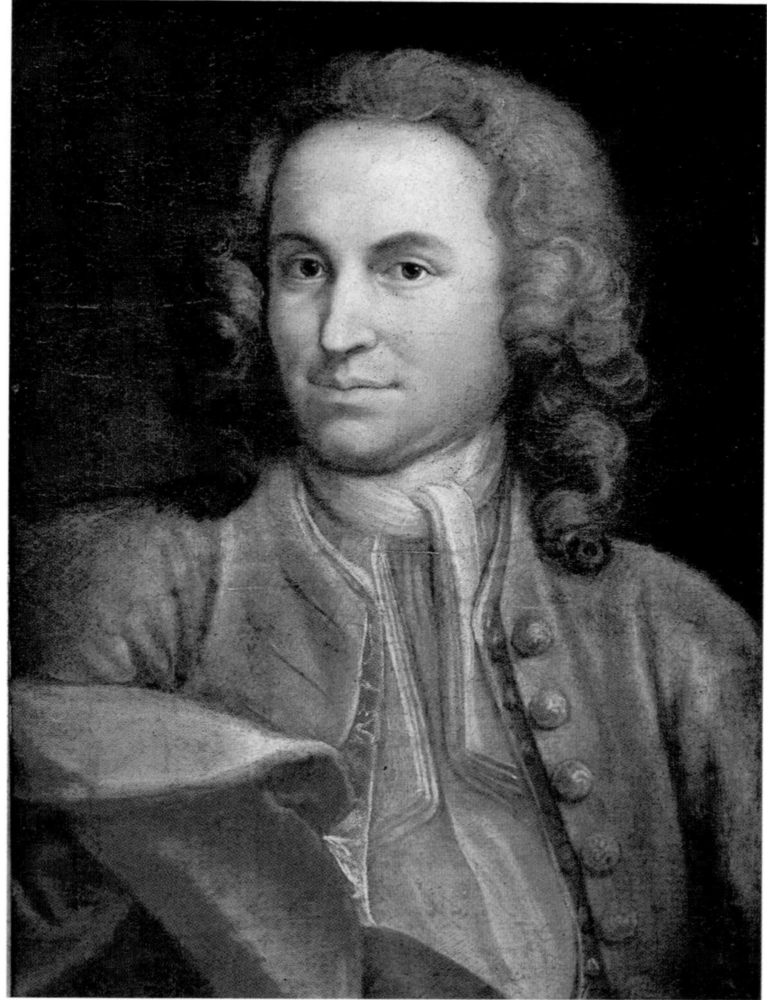

A portrait of Johann Sebastian Bach as a young man

Johann Sebastian Bach was born in the German town of Eisenach in 1685. During his lifetime, J. S. Bach was known more as a great harpsichord player and organist than as a composer. Most of the beautiful music he wrote didn't become popular until many years after he died.

HEINRICH'S
PIZZA
It's Heinrich the pizza man.
His pizza's the worst in the land.
He tops them with seaweed and rubberbands
and anything else from his old garbage cans!
I hate these Bach family reunions.

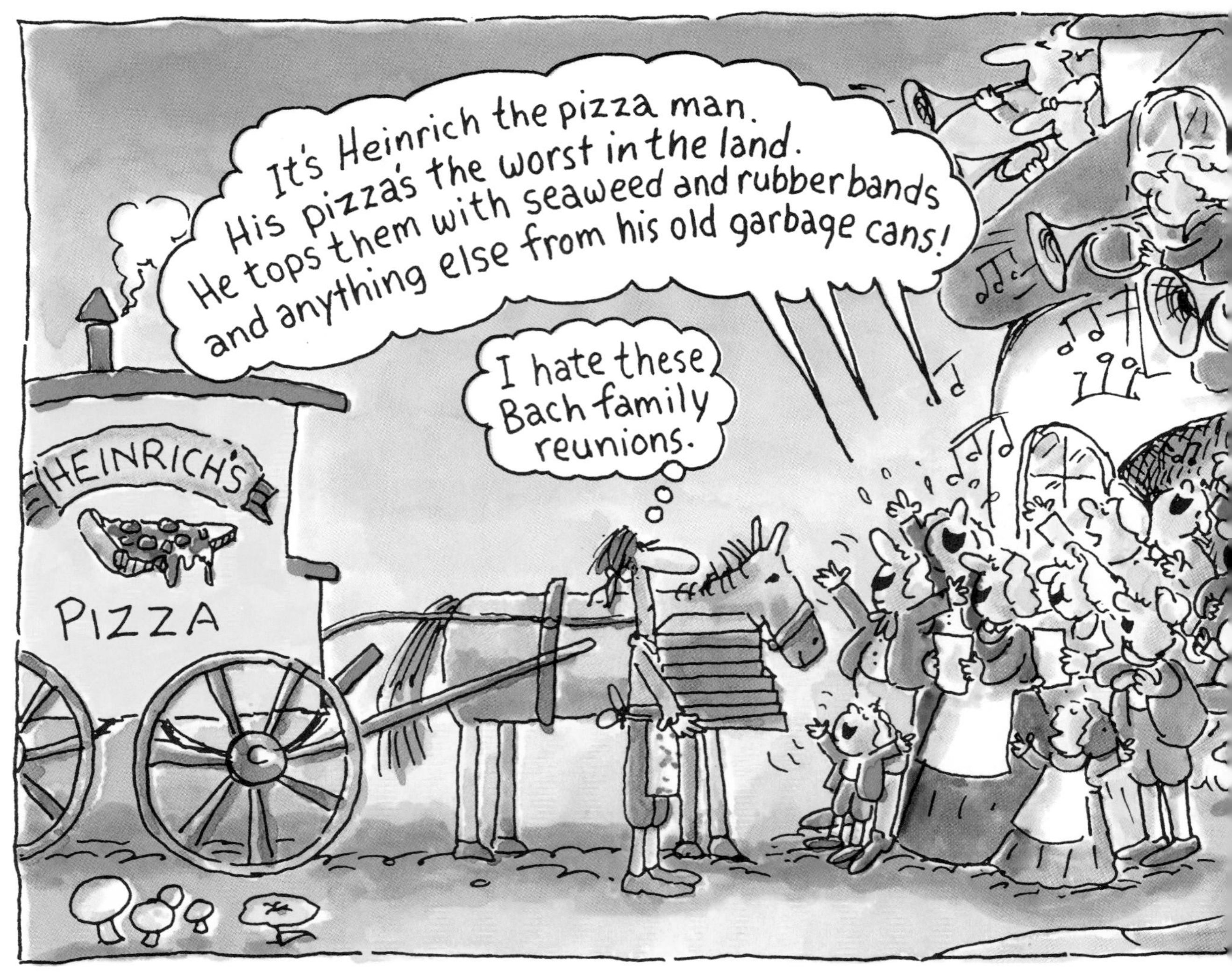

Johann Sebastian Bach came from a large family of musicians. More than seventy of his uncles, cousins, brothers, and other relatives made their livings as musicians, choirmasters, and composers. There were so many musical Bachs in Germany that in some areas, being a

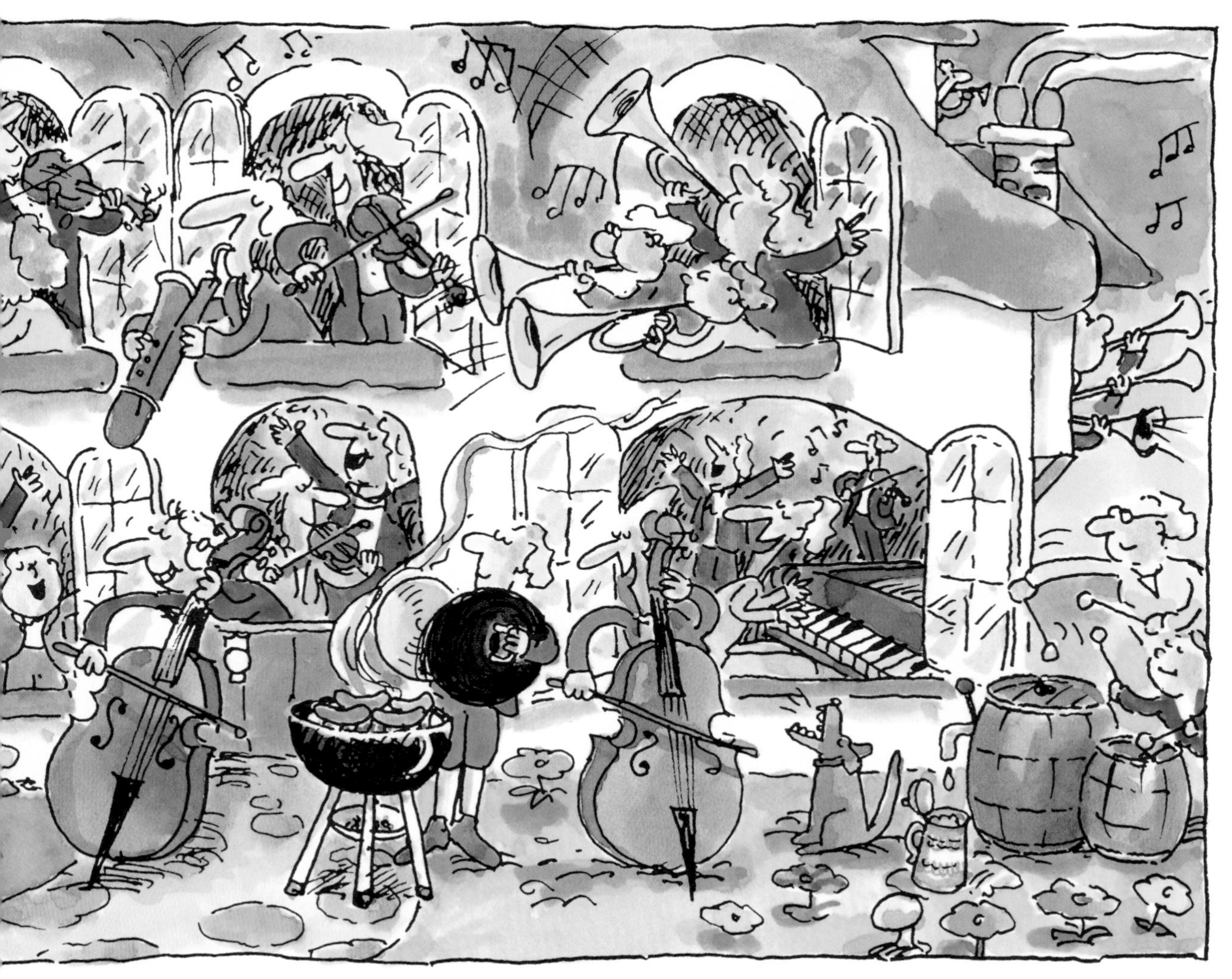

Bach meant the same thing as being a musician.

Every year, members of the Bach family got together for a reunion. They had a great time playing their favorite music and then making up funny songs that kept them laughing for hours.

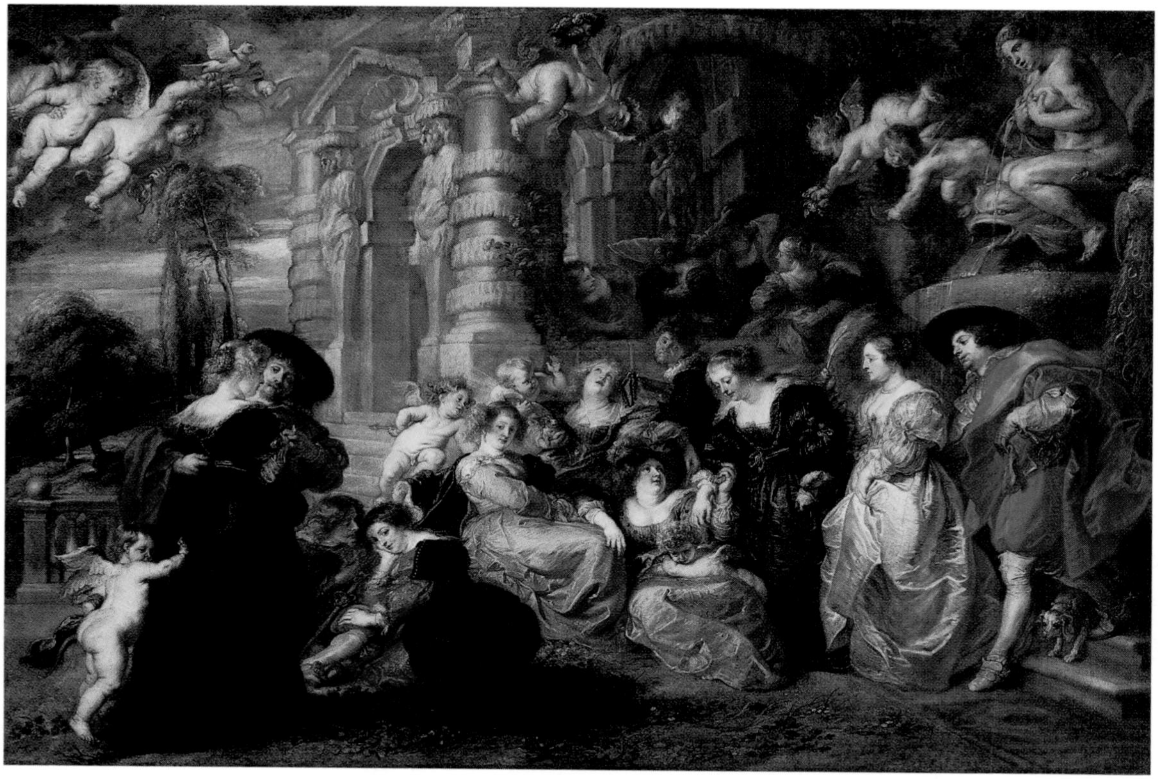

Johann Sebastian Bach played and composed his music during a time known as the Baroque period. In the 1600s and 1700s, everything in Europe seemed to have a grand, fancy, and decorative feeling to it. Art and architecture were created to show off the palaces and homes of kings, queens, dukes, and wealthy businessmen.

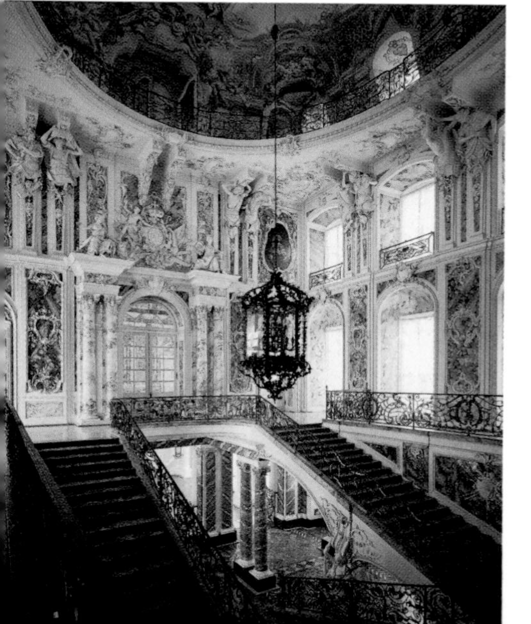

A painting by Baroque artist Peter Paul Rubens (above) and a stairway inside a Baroque German palace (left)

Gee, the new playroom addition looks great! Are you going to paint it next??
No. We usually just cover everything with whipped cream and frosting.

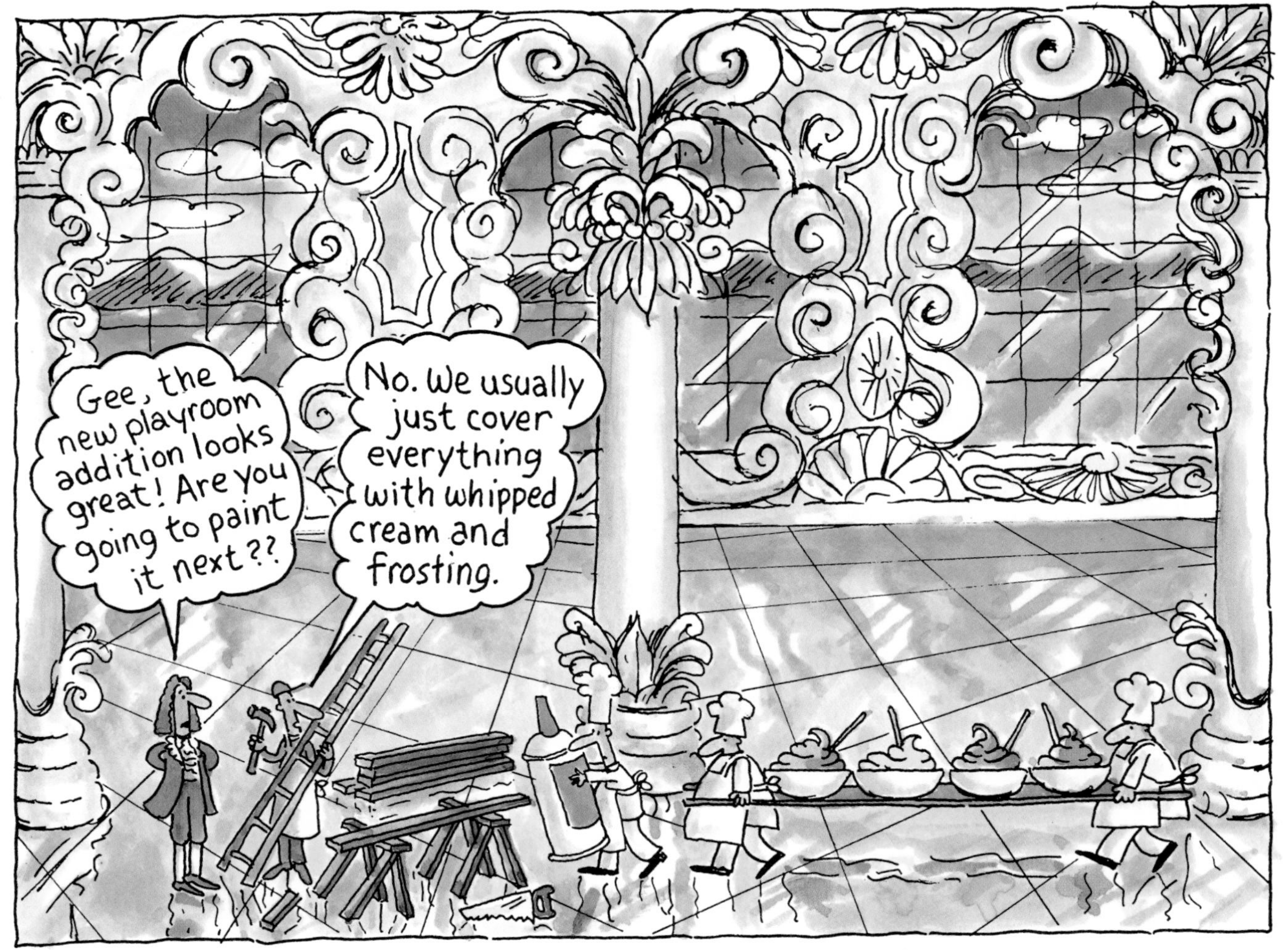

Baroque music also had kind of a grand, decorative feeling. It was often filled with the sounds of voices, violins, trumpets, and flutes, each playing different melodies at the same time. J. S. Bach was an expert at making complicated Baroque pieces sound natural and pleasing.

Wealthy people would listen to their favorite Baroque music at royal court gatherings or at the opera. Regular everyday people could hear wonderful choral and organ music in their local churches.

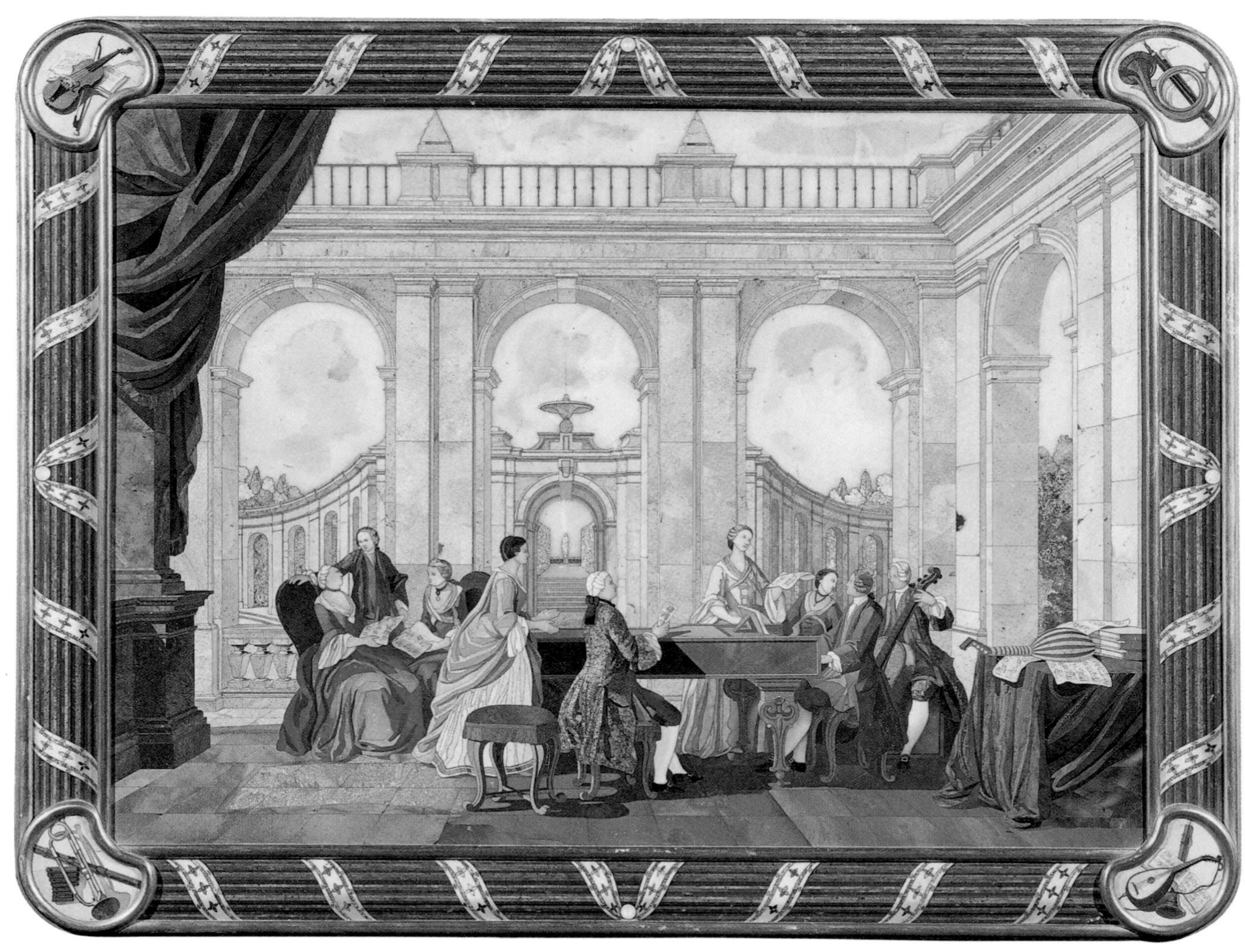

Musicians playing during a European court gathering in the early 1700s

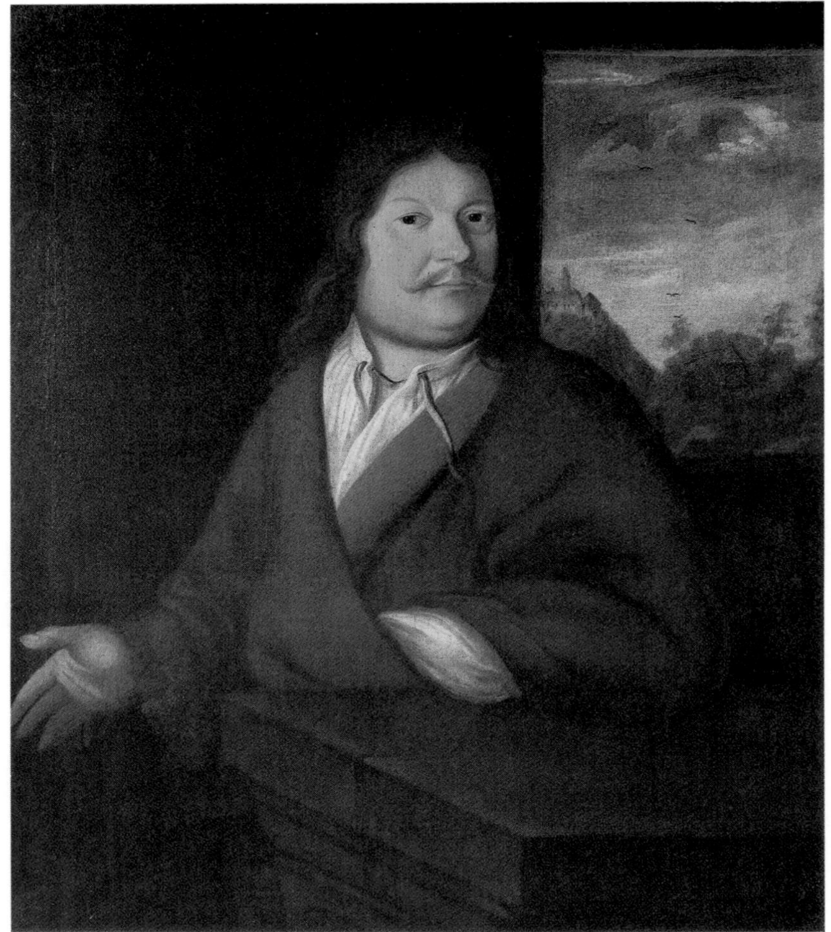

Johann Ambrosius Bach, the father of Johann Sebastian Bach

Town musicians often played at celebrations and special events. J. S. Bach's father was a town musician. He probably taught his son to play the violin and introduced him to other instruments.

When J. S. Bach (who was usually called Sebastian) was nine years old, a very sad thing happened—his mother died. Then, only a year later, his father died, too.

A sad Sebastian Bach went to live with his older brother, Christoph, in the nearby town of Ohrdruf. Christoph Bach was known as an excellent church organist. He not only taught Sebastian to play the harpsichord and organ, but how to tune and fix broken organs.

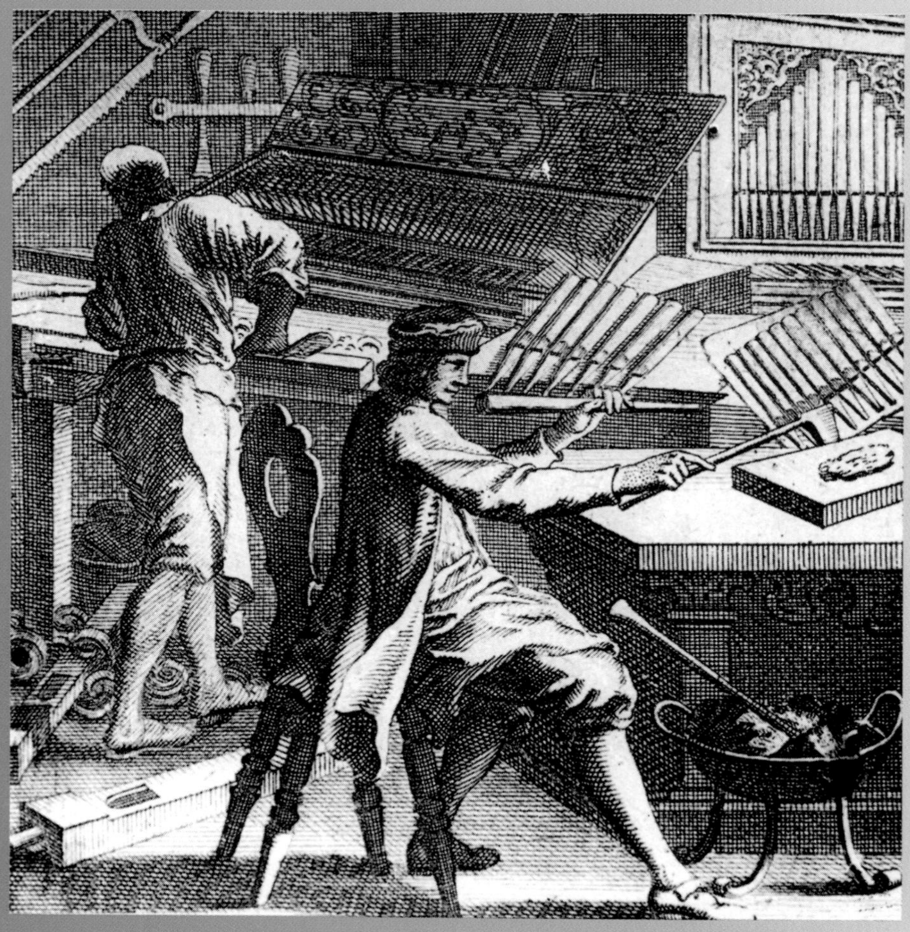

Organs being built and repaired in the early 1700s

Ah... I'll be right back. I have to check something with my brother. It's my first job, you know.

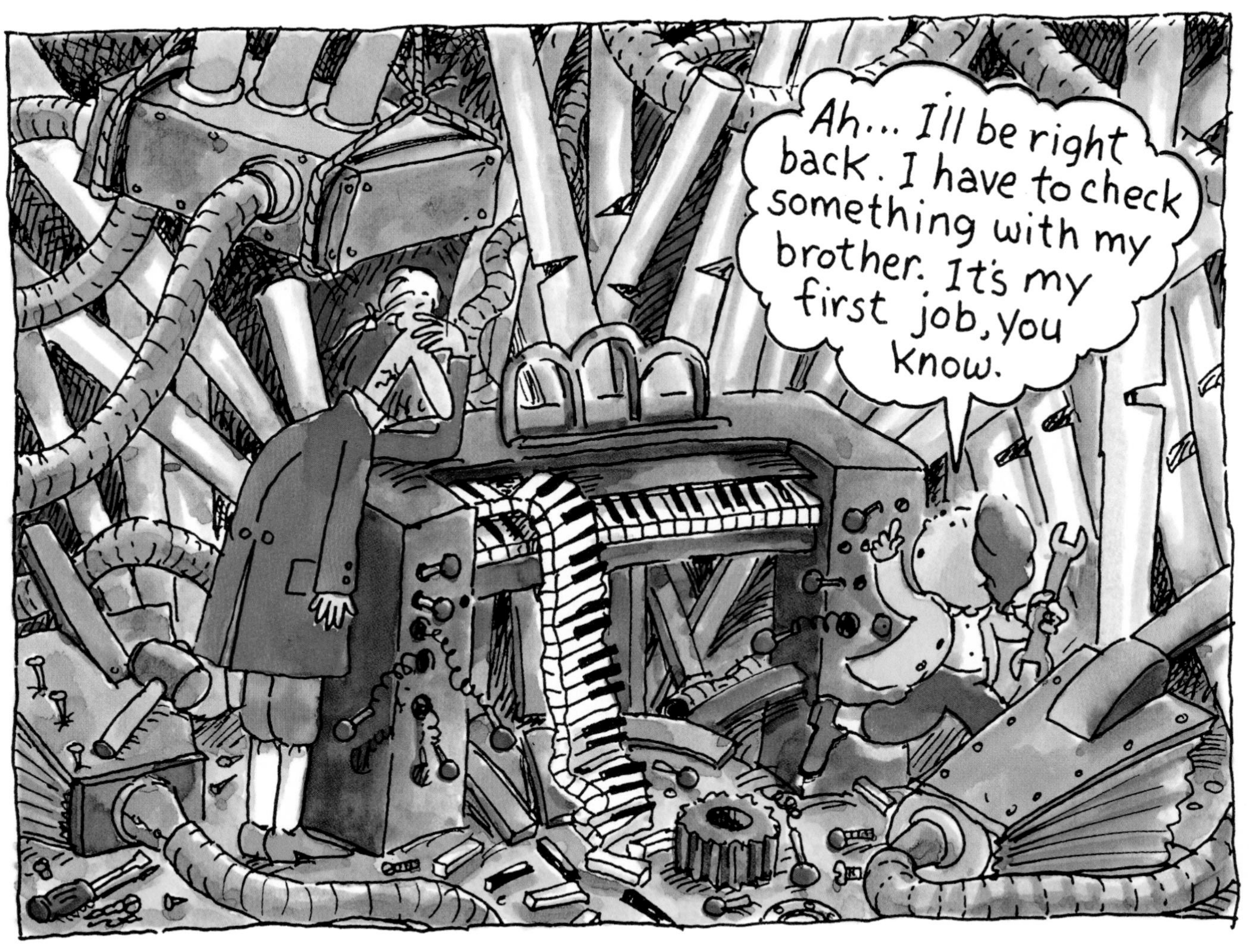

Johann Sebastian Bach tested and repaired organs in different towns around Germany. It was one of the ways he made extra money throughout his life.

When Sebastian was fifteen years old, he left his brother's home to look for a job. He traveled two hundred miles on foot to the town of Luneburg. There he attended school and became a member of the church choir.

This was the beginning of many trips Sebastian would take during his life. He was always looking for the best music job he could get. Sometimes, his music jobs came along with chores that weren't very pleasant. When he was seventeen years old, Sebastian got a great job as a violinist in the royal court at Celle, Germany. But as part of the job, he also had to remove slop from the kitchen every morning!

Our new violinist is very talented.
So is our new organist. He can peel a whole sack of potatoes in less than 3 minutes.

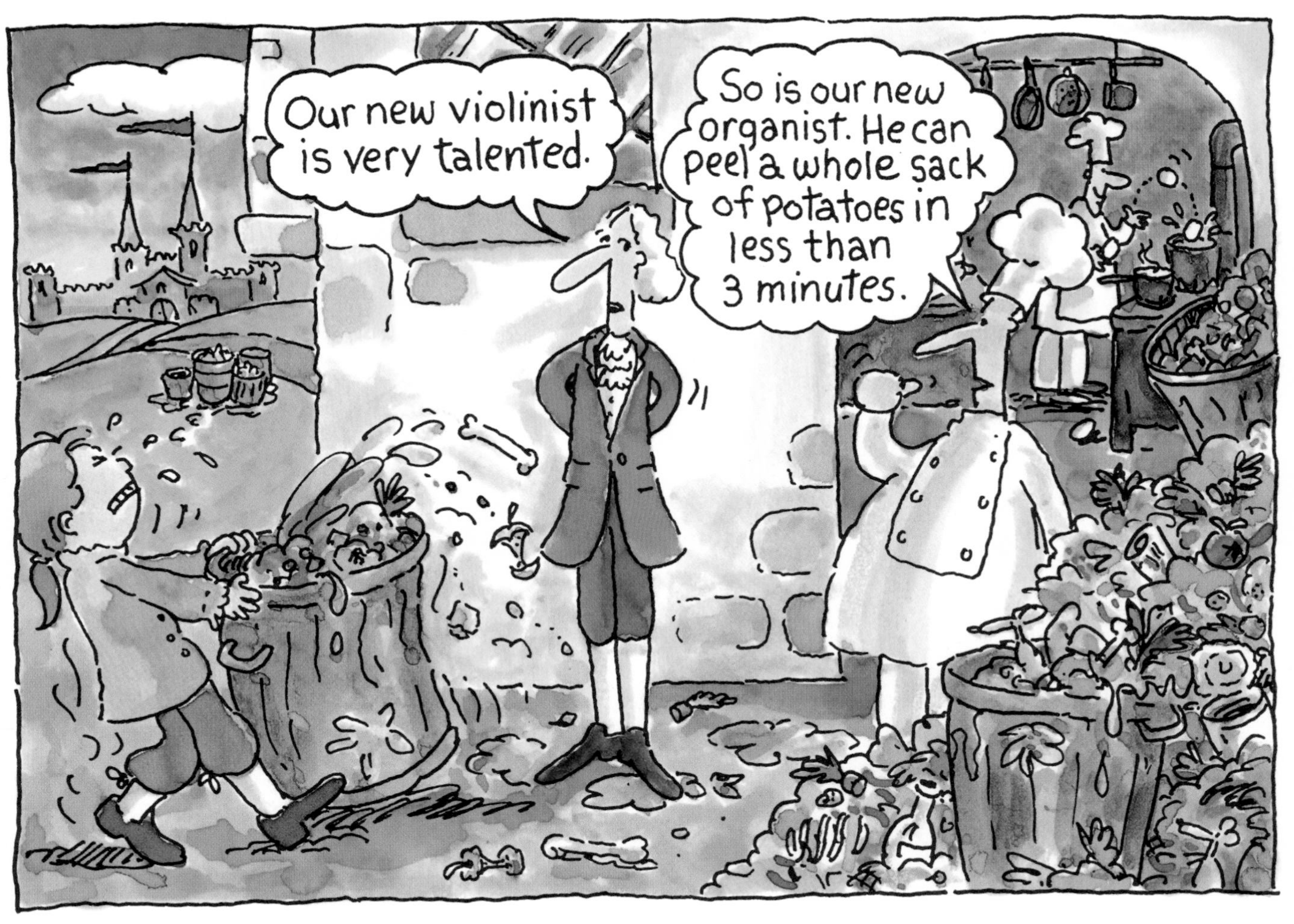

As he moved to different towns, working as a choirmaster (a person who leads a choir), musician, or church organist, J. S. Bach learned more and more about music.

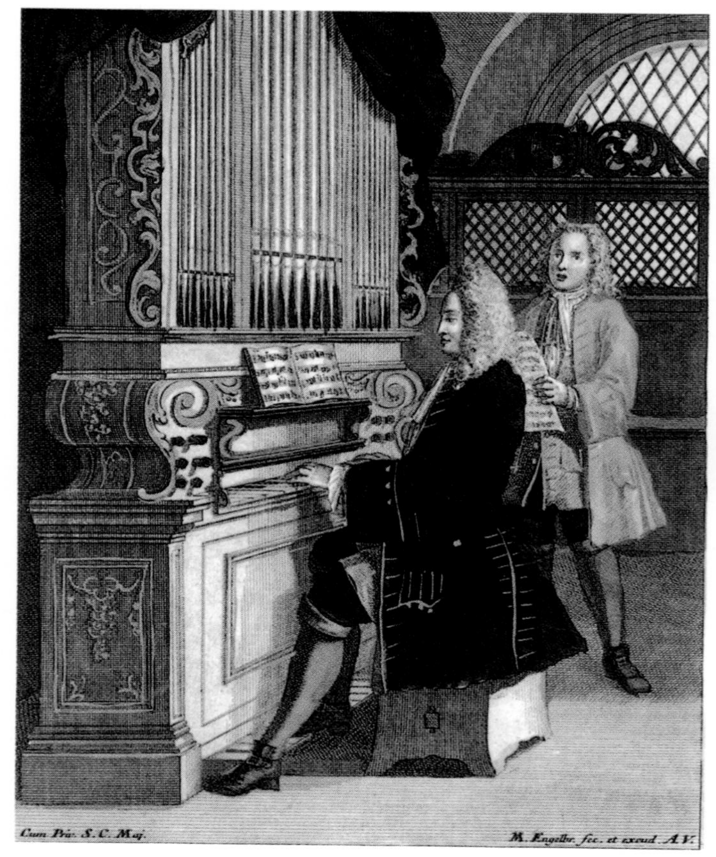


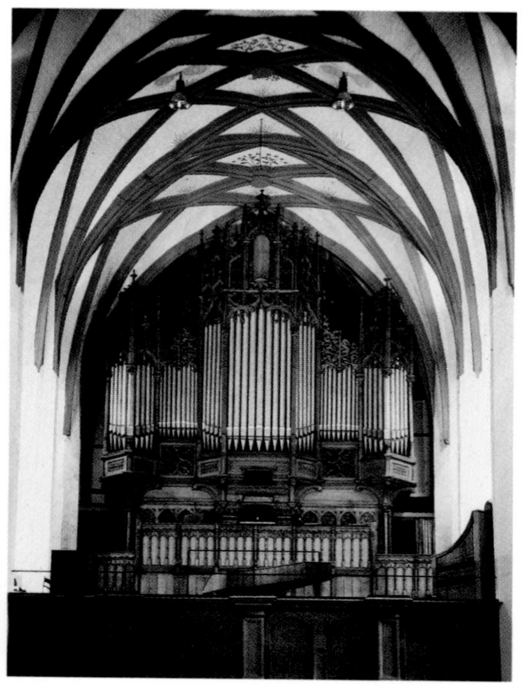

A 17th-century organist (left) and a photograph of one of the organs played by Bach (right)

Johann Sebastian Bach took side trips, too. He wanted to listen to well-known organists and composers to get ideas for his own music. On one trip, he heard a famous organist named Dietrich Buxtehude play. Sebastian was inspired by Buxtehude's animated and imaginative music. Soon Sebastian started creating new and exciting music in his own style.

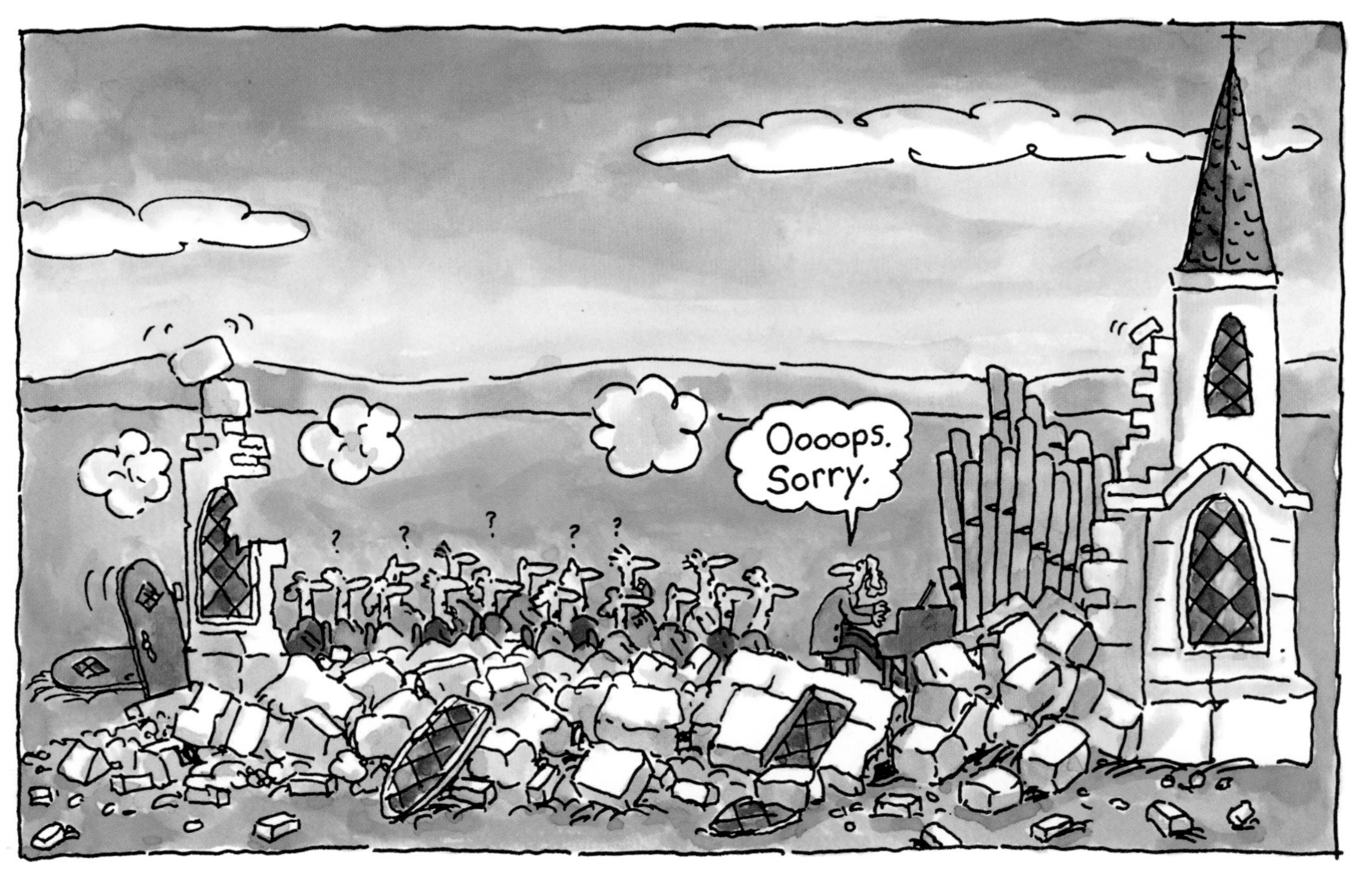


One of Bach's most famous organ compositions during this time is called *Toccata and Fugue in D Minor*. This piece is filled with big, powerful sounds. It had an energy and force that had never been heard before. Many of J. S. Bach's mighty organ pieces have been known to cause church rafters and windows to shake!

Johann Sebastian Bach was a very religious person. He belonged to the Lutheran Church. One important type of musical piece he wrote for church services is called a cantata. A cantata features mainly voices. It usually has a lead singer and a choir accompanied by an orchestra. J.S. Bach wrote hundreds of cantatas. In each one you can feel his love for God. These beautiful works were a very important part of the Lutheran church service.

Bach's cantatas usually used hymn tunes, called chorales, that most people knew and loved.

Mom! How much longer?!!
About 4 hours and 55 minutes. Now settle down, and try to relax.

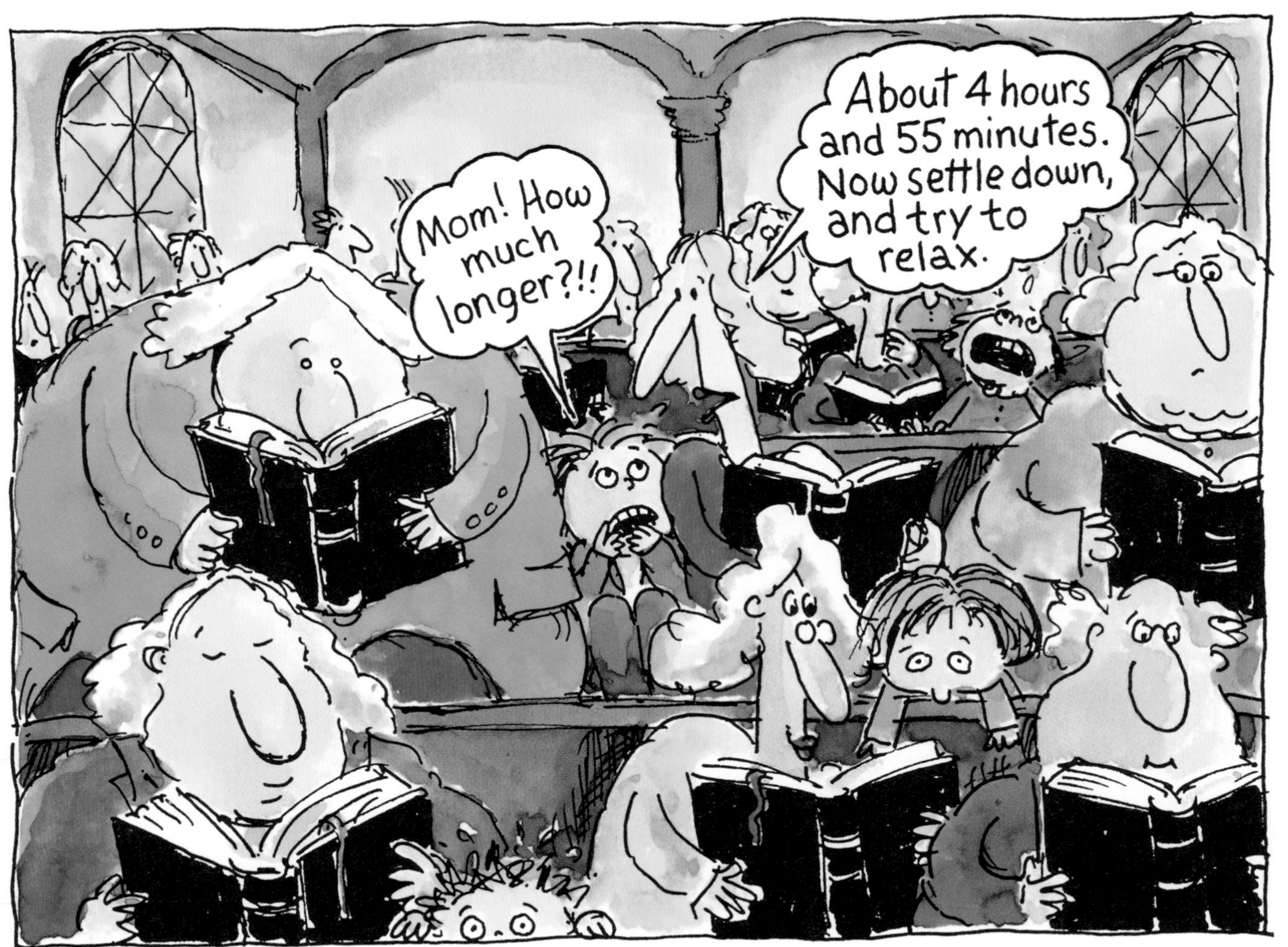

In J. S. Bach's time, a church service could last for five hours or more! People depended on cantata music to keep them interested and awake.

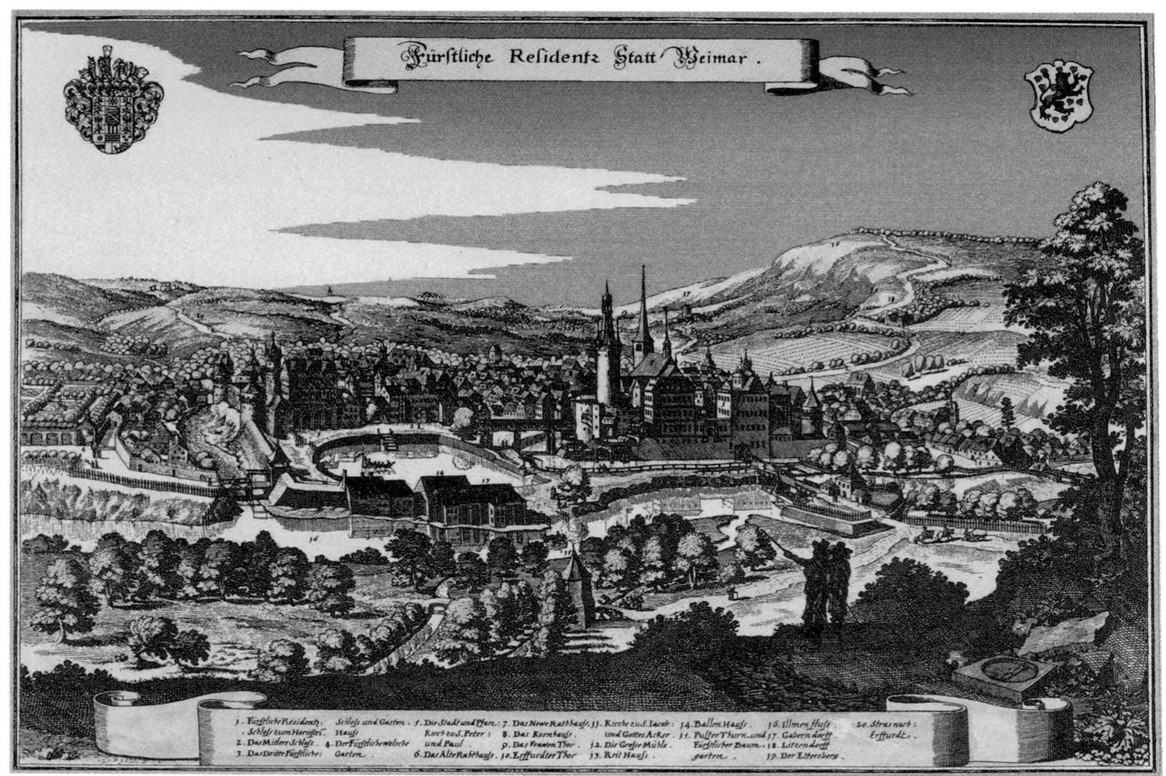


Weimar as it looked during Bach's time

It wasn't long before J. S. Bach became well known for his remarkable talent as an organist and composer of church music. This made it easier for him to find better jobs. When Sebastian was working as an organist in the town of Muhlhausen, Germany, he met and fell in love with Maria Barbara Bach, a distant cousin. Maria was happy to travel around with her husband and raise their family.

In 1708, Sebastian got an excellent job in the court of Duke Wilhelm Ernst of Saxe-Weimar. Bach wrote some of his most important organ works there. Unfortunately, after a few years, Sebastian felt the duke was becoming too bossy. He decided to take a new job at a friendlier court. When the duke heard about Bach's decision, he became angry and had Johann Sebastian Bach thrown in jail for a whole month!

What are you guys in for?
MURDER!
ROBBERY!!
Smuggling bratwurst across the border!!
Switching jobs.

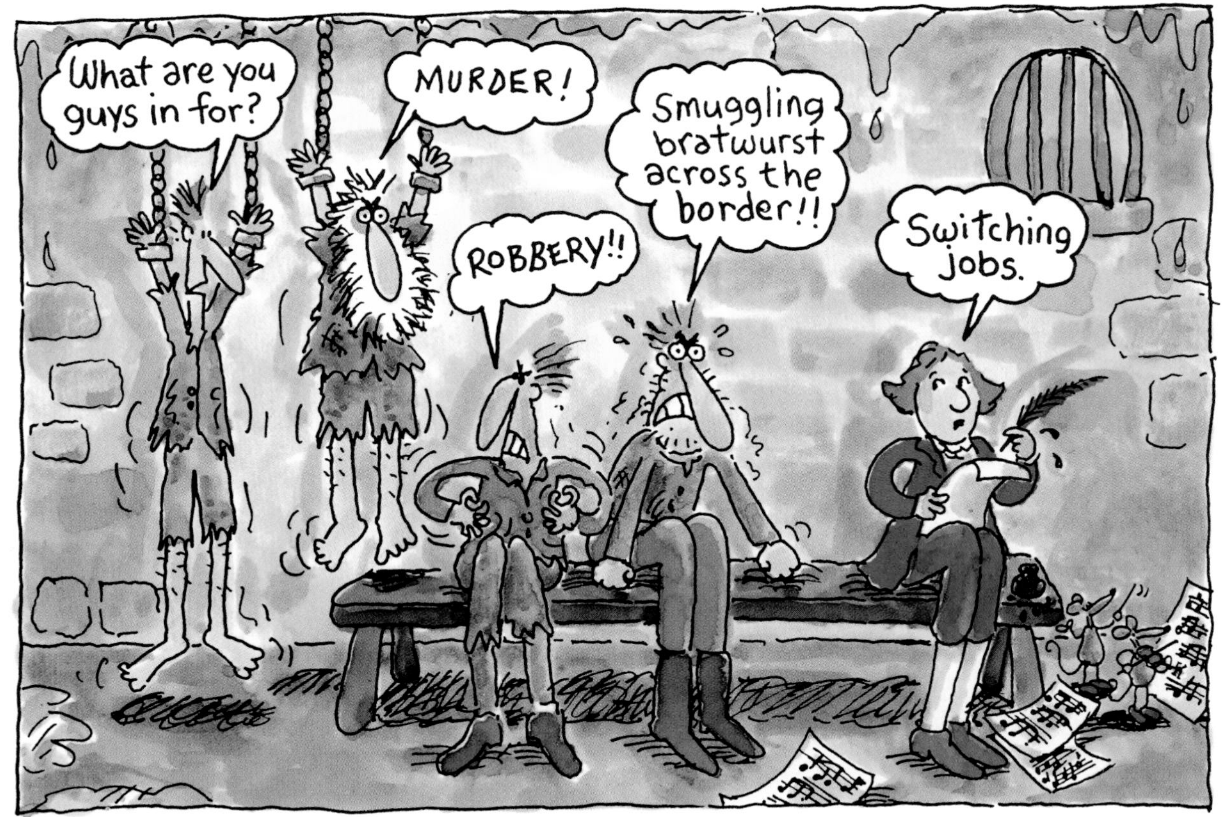

Being in jail was a very depressing experience for Johann Sebastian Bach. He couldn't wait to get out and start his new job with Prince Leopold of Cöthen, Germany. Sebastian and the prince got along really well. Sebastian composed mainly instrumental music for the prince. He also wrote the first book of *The Well-Tempered Clavier*, and *The Little Organ Book*. These keyboard works are still played by music students today.

After six happy years in Prince Leopold's court, things quickly changed for the worse. First, Sebastian's wife, Maria, died. Then the prince got married, and his new wife didn't care for music at all.

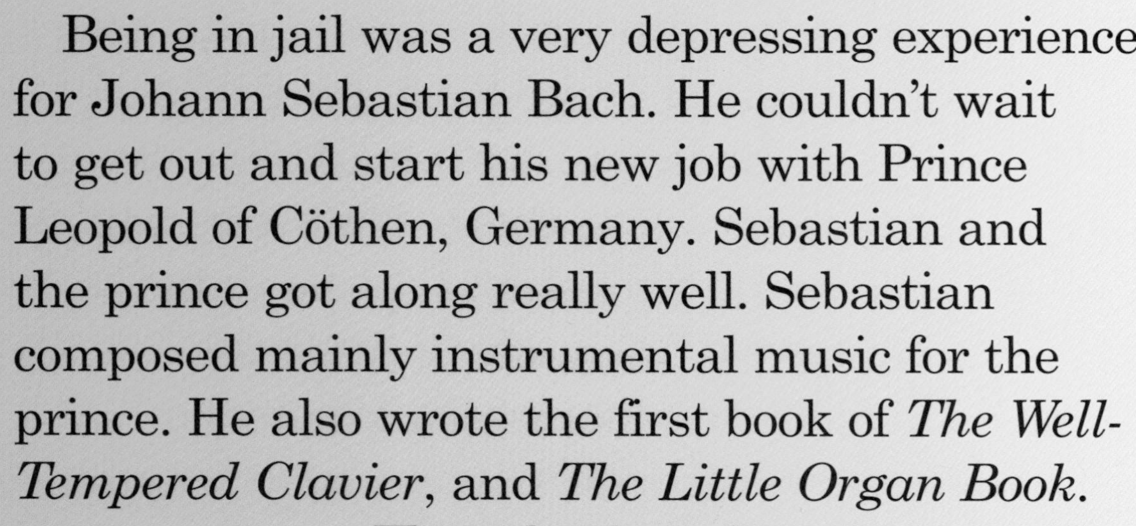

Prince Leopold of Cöthen

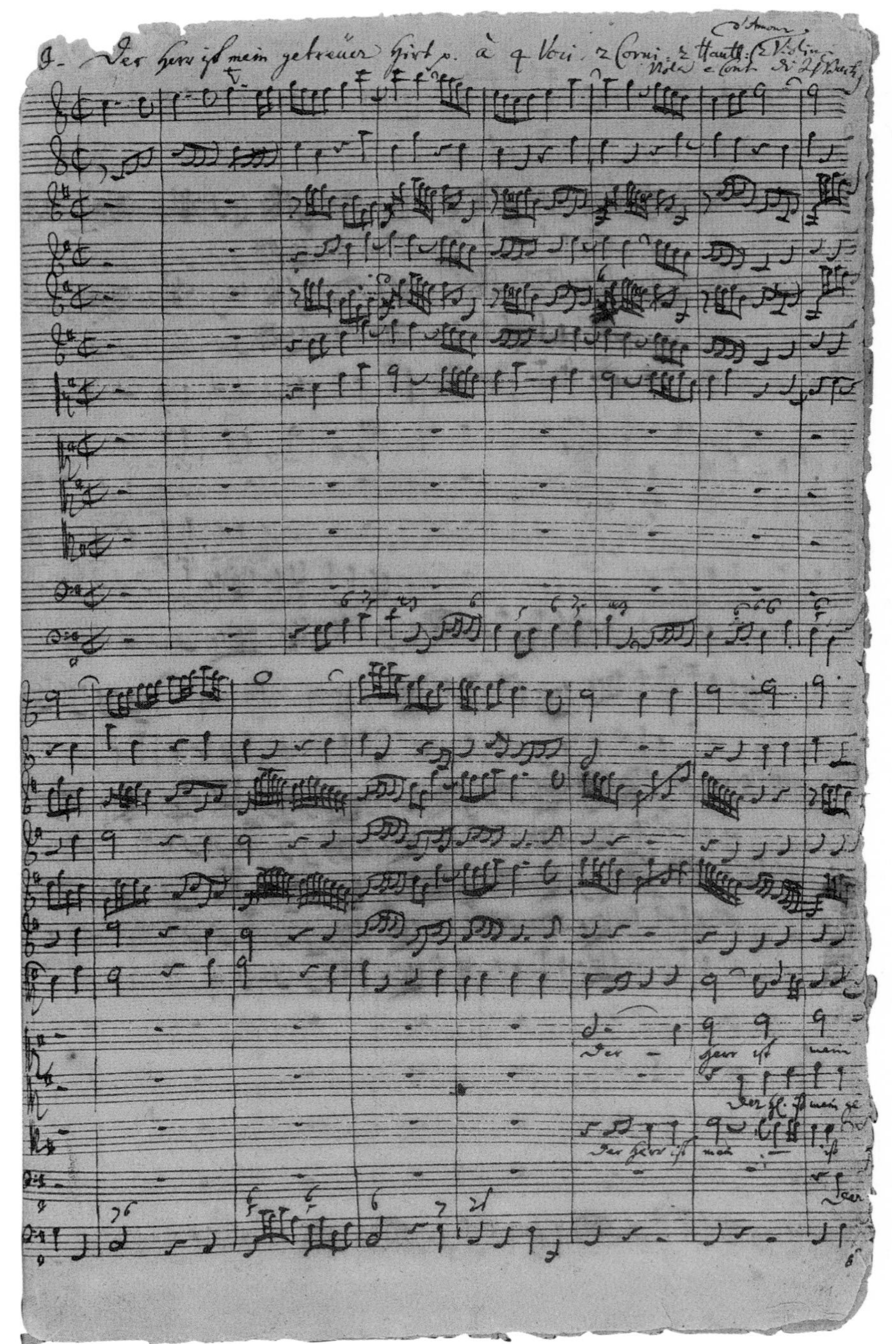

A page from an original handwritten piece of music by J.S. Bach

Soon, the prince started losing interest in music too. Sebastian felt it was time to move on and look for a new job again.

Before he left Prince Leopold's court, J. S. Bach wrote a set of his most famous and popular works—the *Brandenburg Concertos*. A concerto is a musical piece in which one instrument, or a small group of instruments, stands out from the rest of the orchestra. It's a good way for an excellent musician to show off his or her talent. In the *Brandenburg Concertos*, trumpets, violins, oboes, flutes, harpsichords, or cellos play along with a larger orchestra to make up some of the best "feeling-happy" music ever.

Doc, I've been feeling grouchy lately!!!
Try listening to 6 Brandenburg concertos, and call me in the morning.

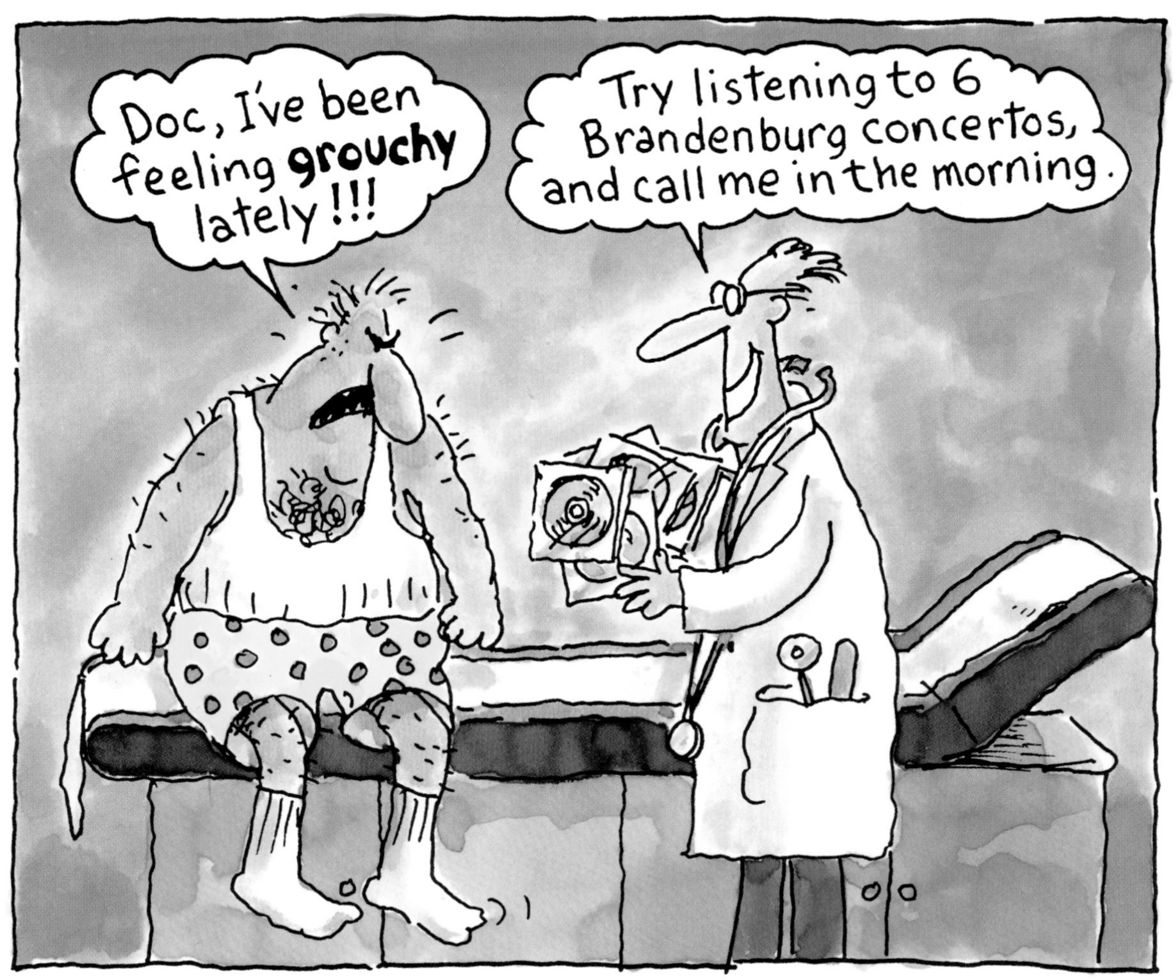

If you are in a grouchy or sad mood, these concertos are almost guaranteed to make you feel better. The *Brandenburg Concertos* are filled with beautiful musical sounds that are sometimes relaxing and peaceful, and sometimes bursting with joy. You can almost imagine yourself being at a royal event in some duke or king's palace when you listen to these pieces.

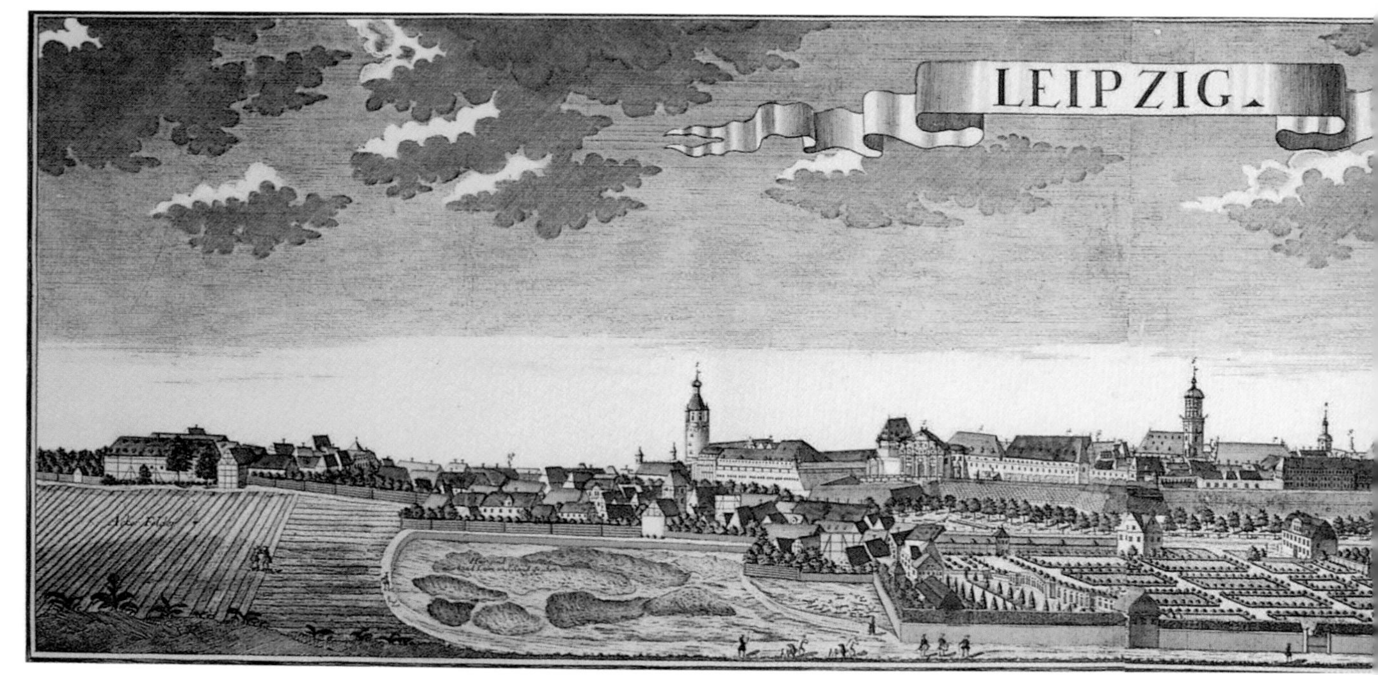


In 1723, J. S. Bach accepted a job as director of music in the historic city of Leipzig, Germany. This was probably Sebastian's busiest time. He was responsible for composing and directing music for four churches, a school choir, a university choir, and any music the city might need for special events.

Sebastian had remarried in 1721. His new wife's name was Anna Magdalena. Anna Magdalena and Sebastian ended up having thirteen children. With four children from his first marriage, Sebastian was very busy taking care of a large family.

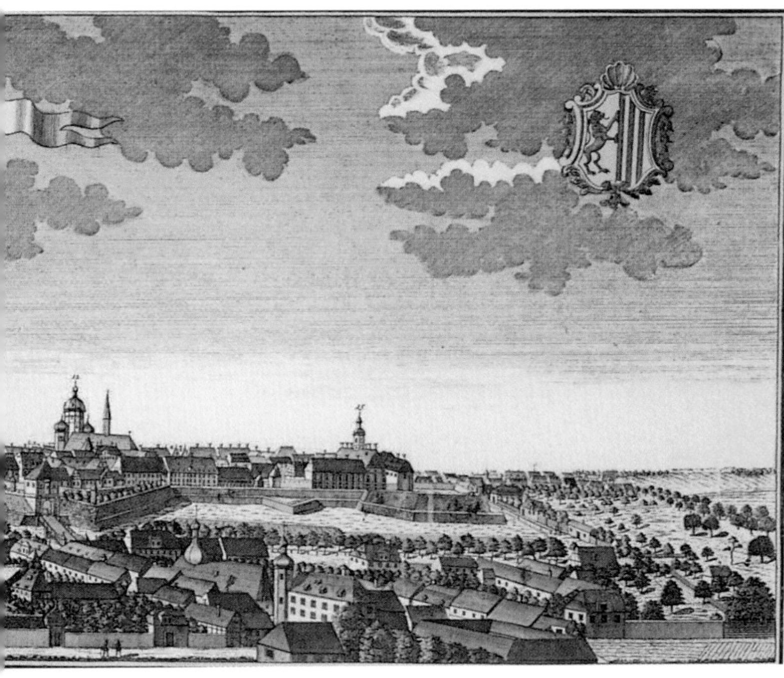

In 1723, Bach became Director of Church Music for the city of Leipzig, Germany.

Johann Sebastian Bach and his family

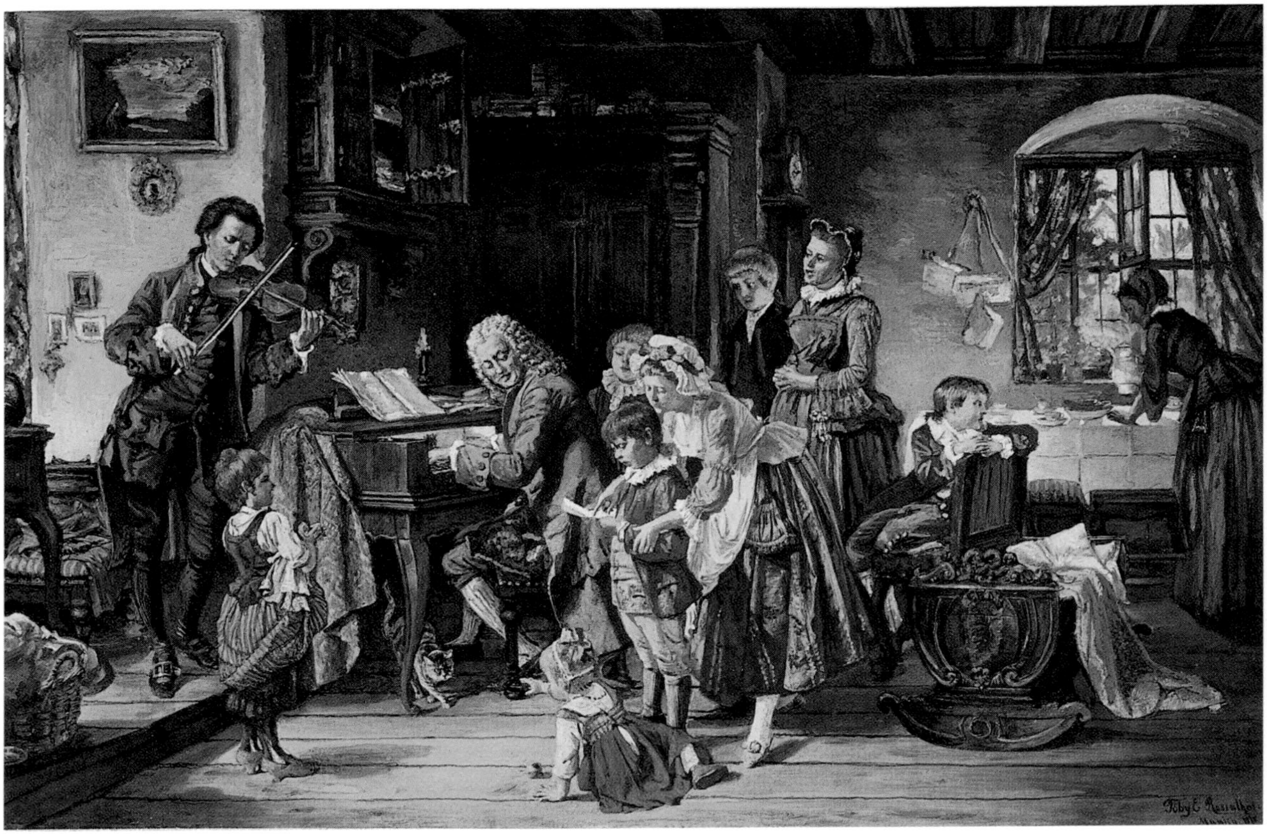

Is everyone ready to practice their music and do their chores?

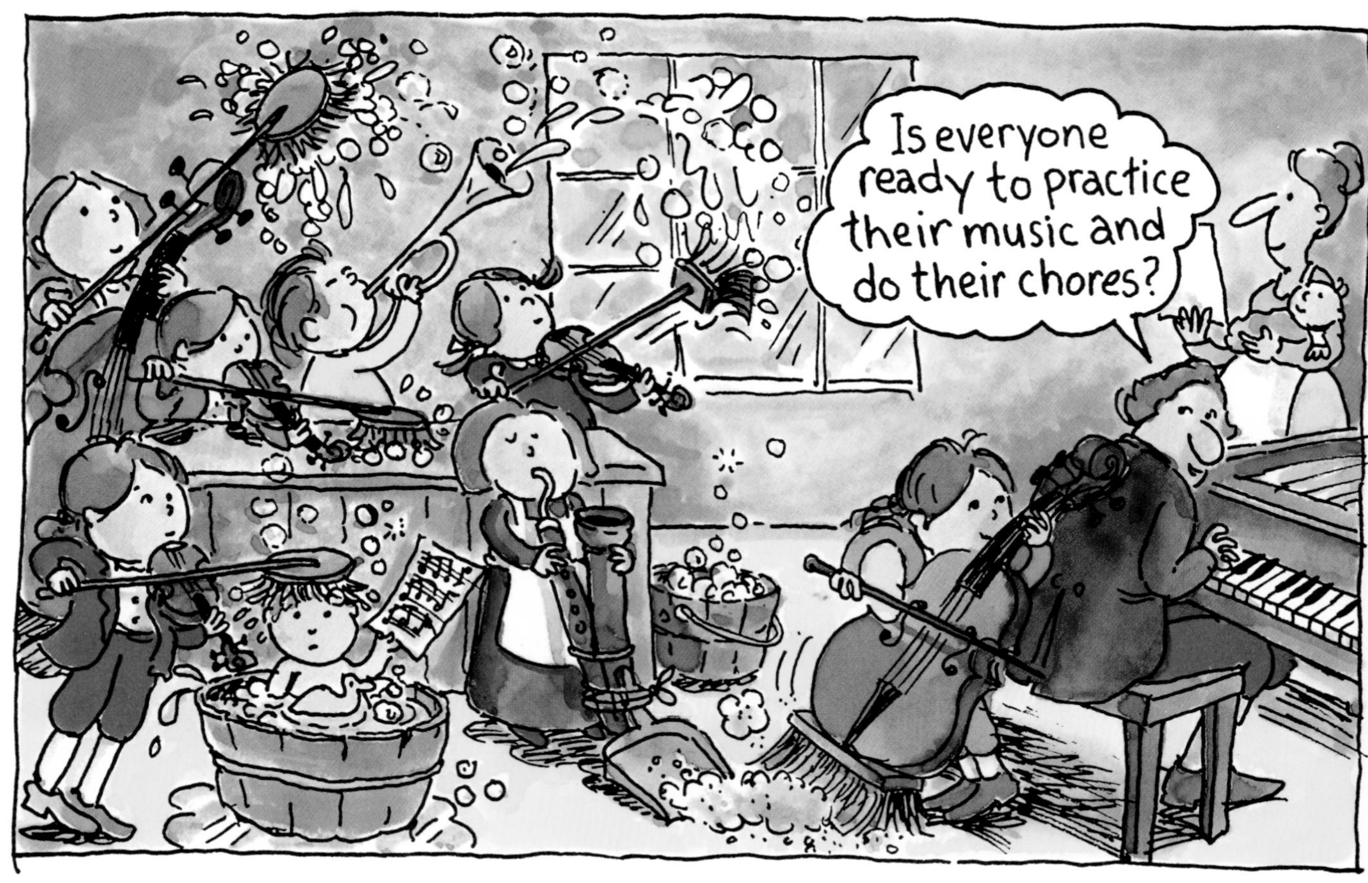

One of the many things Sebastian had to do every week was to write down and make copies of the music he had written for all the choir and orchestra members. This was a really boring job, but Anna Magdalena and their children would often help out. As busy as he was, J. S. Bach always found time for his large family.

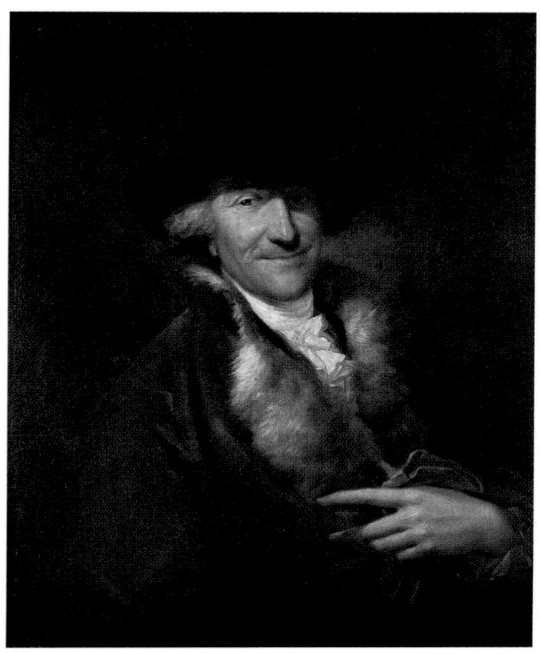

Wilhelm Friedemann Bach

Johann Christian Bach

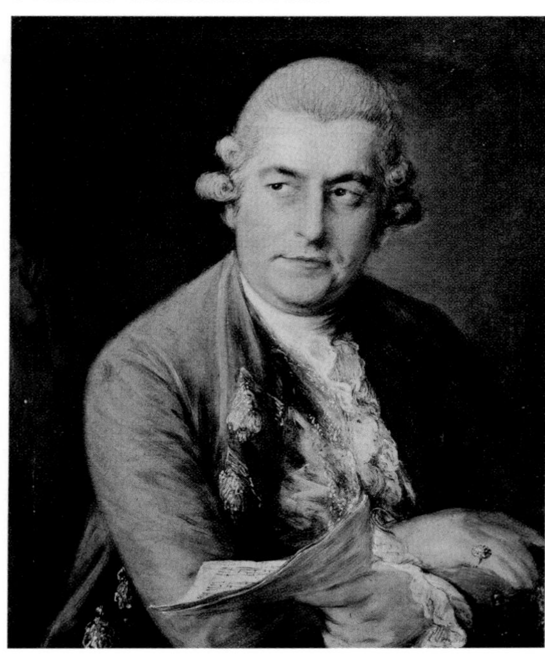

He was a loving father and made sure all his children got good grades, learned to play musical instruments, and helped out around the house. Four of Bach's sons became famous composers and musicians.

C. P. E. Bach

Johann Christoph Friedrich Bach

Johann Sebastian Bach spent twenty-nine years in Leipzig. He composed some of his greatest works there, including the *Goldberg Variations*. These keyboard pieces take you on an amazing sound trip. They start out peacefully, build to a swirling musical whirlwind, and drop you back off where things are nice and calm again.

Another piece from this time, the *St. Matthew Passion*, is filled with heavenly sounds and shows how Bach could put his deepest religious feelings into a work. And the joyful *Christmas Oratorio* has some of the biggest and cheeriest trumpet and horn sounds you'll ever hear!

I WISH TO HOLD THEE TIGHT, BABY!!!
Oooooooooh YEAH!!!
Bach, have you noticed there seems to be a new trend in music these days?
I've noticed.

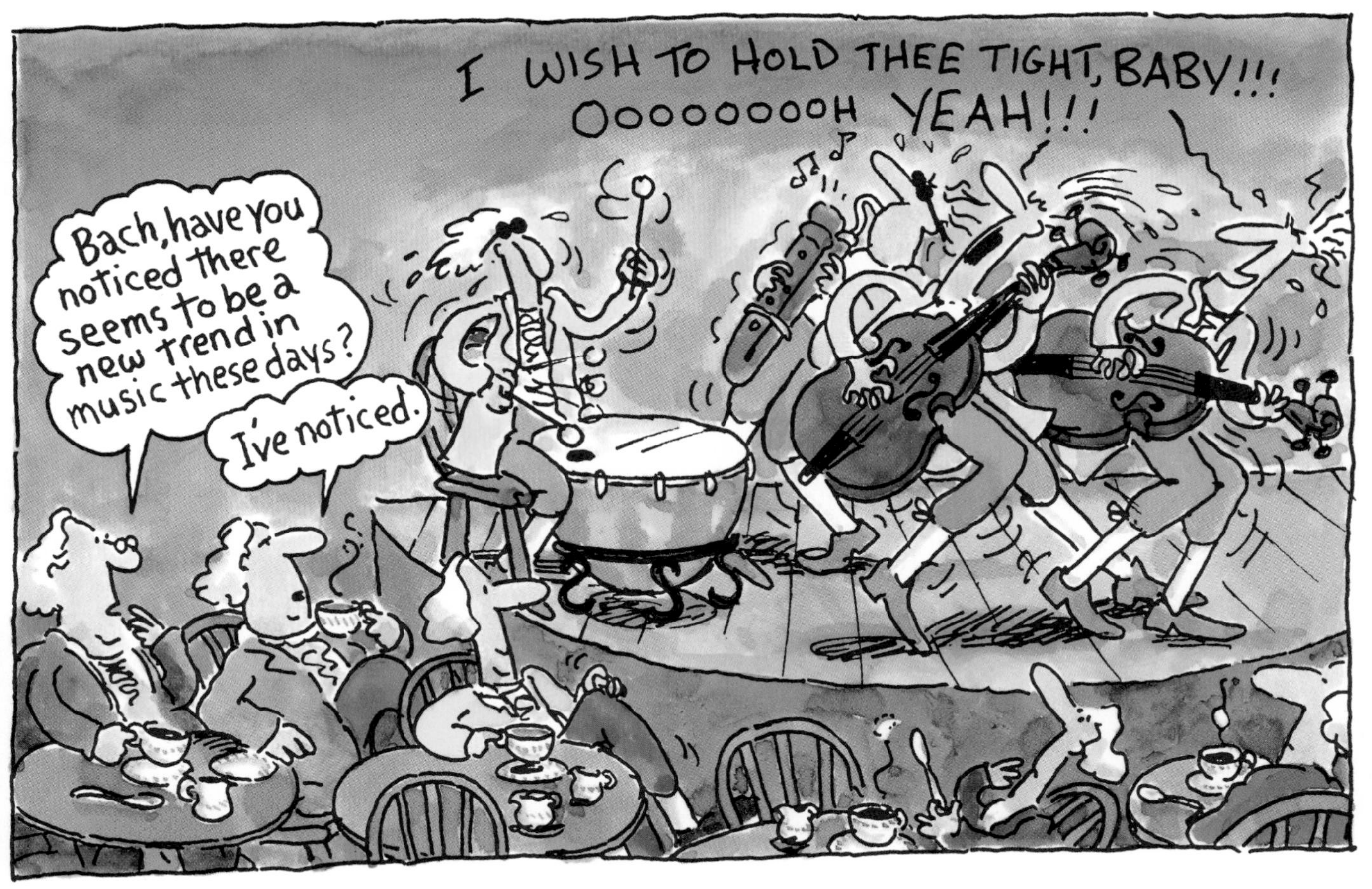

Later in J. S. Bach's life, musical tastes began to change. People were growing tired of what they thought were big, complicated Baroque sounds. They wanted music that was simpler and lighter. Bach heard some of the latest music of the day in coffee houses around Leipzig, where college students and musicians traveling through town sometimes played popular new music.

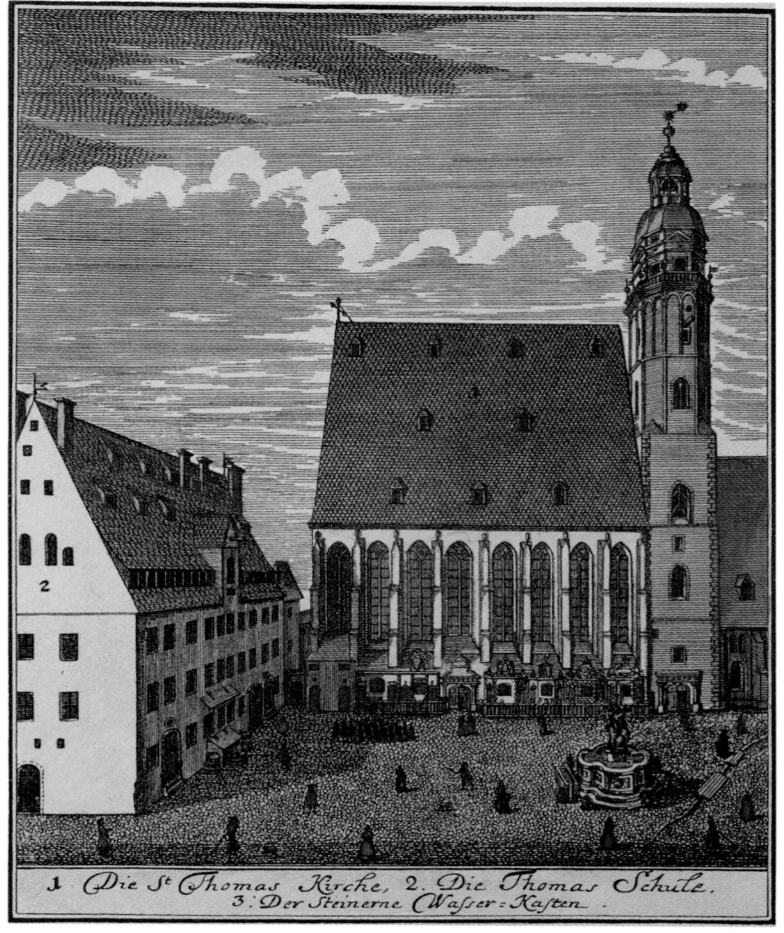


The Thomaskirche, one of the four churches Bach directed music for in Leipzig

Even though Johann Sebastian Bach knew things were changing musically, he decided to stick with his favorite Baroque style. Some people criticized him for being old-fashioned. In Leipzig, it seemed like Bach was always being given a hard time, especially from his bosses. J. S. Bach had dozens of bosses. Most of them had very little understanding of music.

Bach always had trouble getting raises or money for necessary music equipment. Members of the town council thought Sebastian wasn't working hard enough. The principal of the church school thought music was a waste of time for his students. And the head of the university thought Bach was directing the choir poorly!

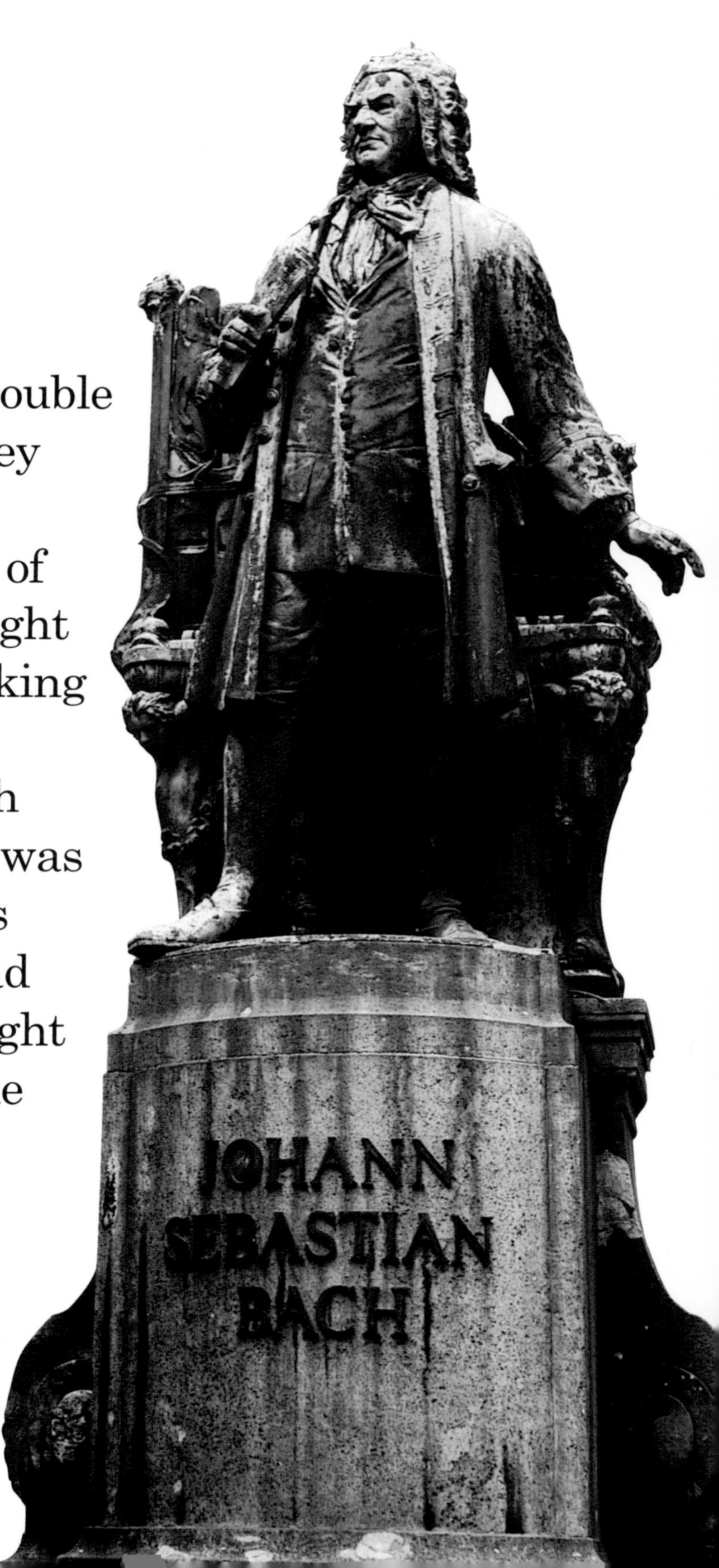


A statue of Johann Sebastian Bach in front of the Thomaskirche in Leipzig

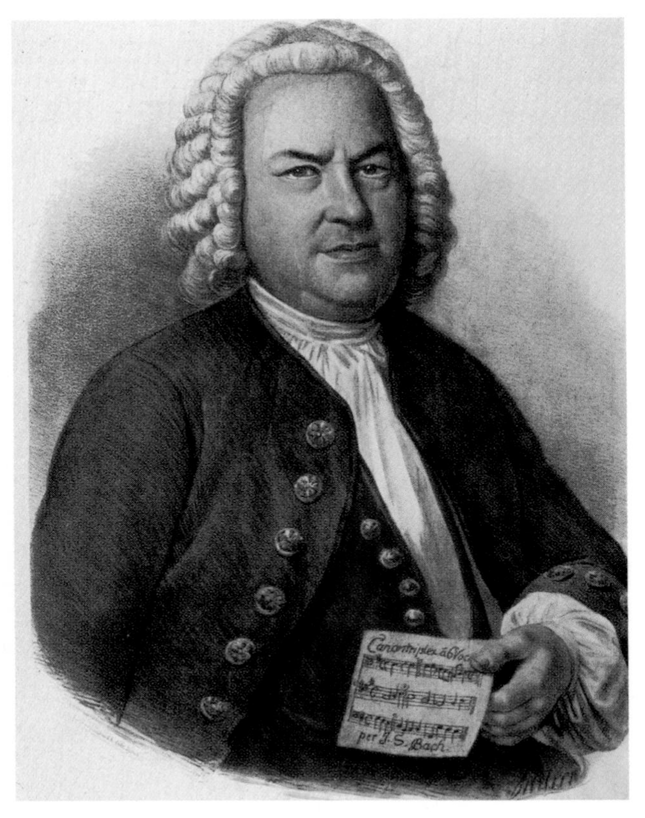


A portrait of Johann Sebastian Bach holding a piece of his own music

Johann Sebastian Bach always stood up for his rights, though. He often ignored silly complaints. When he died in 1750, he had composed some of the world's most beautiful music ever, whether his bosses liked it or not!

It's easy to hear Bach's great music. It's often played on the radio on classical music stations. There are hundreds of tapes and compact discs of his work, too. Also, many neighborhood churches put on free Bach concerts throughout the year.